Men'sHealth
Plant-Based Eating
(THE DIET THAT **CAN** INCLUDE MEAT)

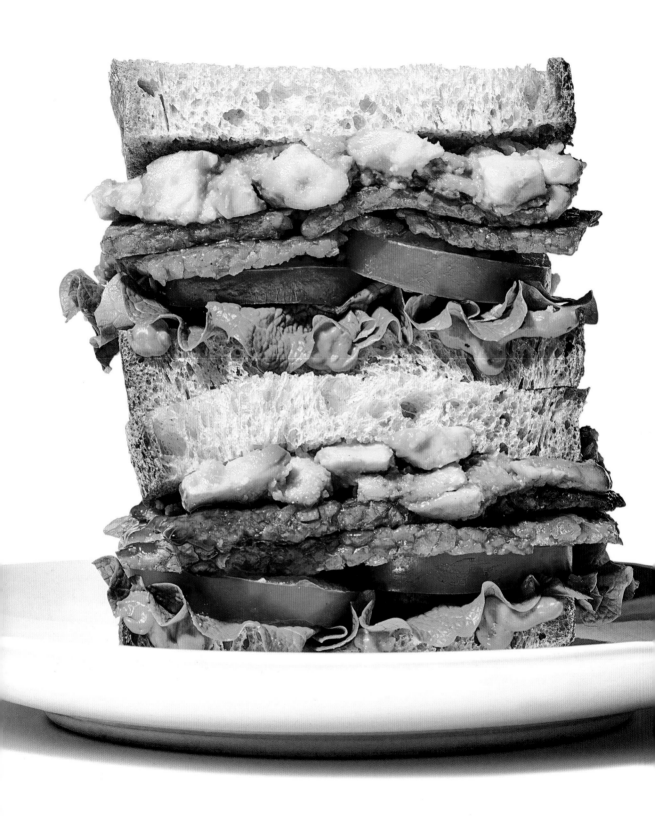

Men'sHealth
Plant-Based
Eating
(THE DIET THAT **CAN** INCLUDE MEAT)

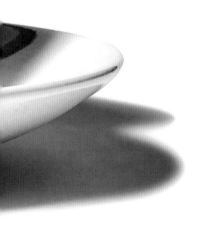

FOREWORD BY
**BRIAN ST. PIERRE,
M.S., R.D., C.S.C.S.**

INTRODUCTION BY
PAUL KITA
FOOD & NUTRITION
EDITOR, *MEN'S HEALTH*

**HEARST
HOME**

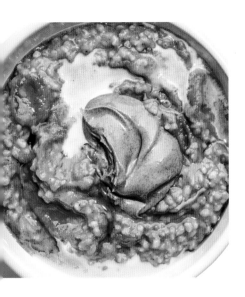

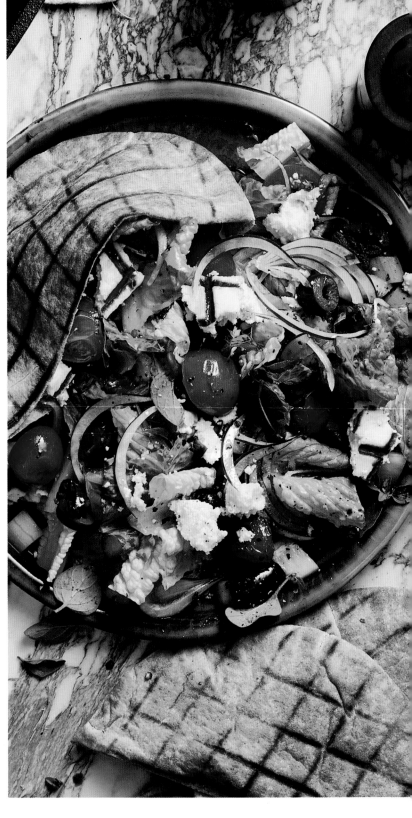

Contents

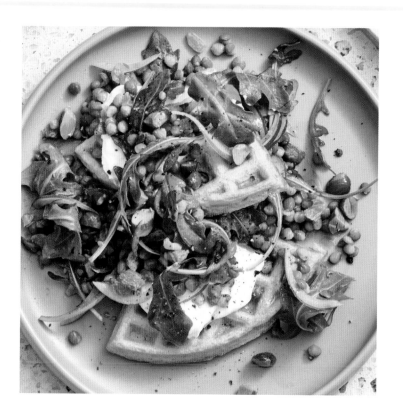

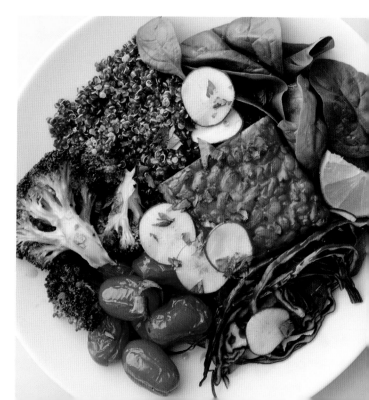

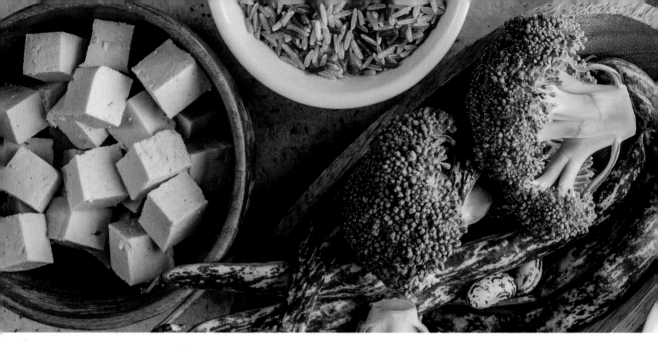

FOREWORD

As a dietitian and director of nutrition at Precision Nutrition, I have worked with my team to teach the concept of a "plant-based" diet for more than a decade to more than 175,000 clients. We've noticed a steady growth in recognition and interest in plant-based eating over that time, and that interest has increased dramatically in the past few years.

Plant-based diets have exploded in popularity, in part due to recent movies like *Forks Over Knives*, *What the Health*, and *The Game Changers*. Yet with each new film, the term "plant-based" grows more confusing as different proponents of this way of eating vary in their interpretations, ranging from strict vegans who do not eat any meat or dairy to individuals who practice Meatless Mondays as their nod to eating more vegetables and grains.

In this book, you'll learn what the term "plant-based" actually means and how you can follow a plant-based way of eating that's right for you. At its core, the goal of a plant-based diet is to eat more whole, minimally processed plants, especially vegetables and fruits.

Any gesture, no matter how small, toward including more plants in our diets can make a difference, as eating your fruits and vegetables comes with multiple health benefits such as fighting disease, losing weight, and prolonging life. Yet according to the Centers for Disease Control and Prevention, only 9 percent of American men (15 percent of women) eat the recommended daily amount of fruit (2 cups), and only 7.6 percent of men (11 percent of women) eat the recommended servings of vegetables (3 cups).

But does that mean you have to go meat-free, eat Beyond Meat, and overhaul your intake to become "plant-based?" We argue no. Your diet is not a zero-sum game. Eating more plant-based foods does not mean you have to give up all animal foods such as meat or eggs.

Our experience at Precision Nutrition—coaching pro athletes as well as "regular folks" who have all types of dietary goals, combined with the full body of clinical evidence—has proven to us that there are many ways to eat healthy. This is why we teach an

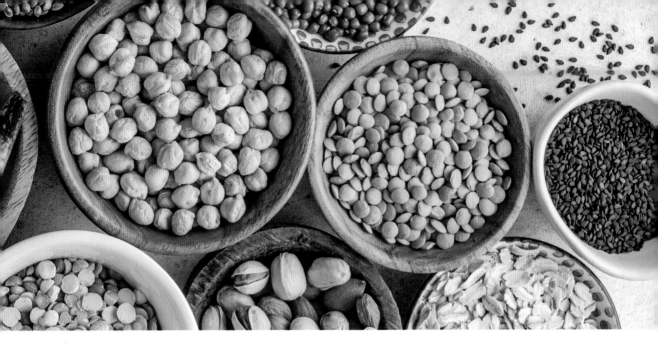

agnostic approach to dietary choices. Both plant-only (done well) or meat-inclusive (done well) can be part of a healthful way of living. You don't have to eat meat to be healthy, strong, or fit. And you don't need to give up meat to be healthy, strong, or fit. It's not a binary either/or proposition.

When you look out across the "diet" landscape, from DASH to Keto, Mediterranean to Paleo, most of the best diets have the same things in common. They emphasize eating an abundance of minimally processed whole foods, including lots of plants, and minimize ultra-processed foods (such as ice cream, chips, and sugar-sweetened beverages). And ultimately, a well done plant-based diet is one that includes lots of plant foods, rather than one that decidedly excludes animal foods. Because it's the inclusion of more and varied plants that improves human health, far more than the exclusion of meat or animal foods.

For me, personally, as a guy who wants to feel good (and look good, I'll be honest), I include lots of whole, minimally processed plants in my diet, along with some meat, dairy, and eggs. And to me, this is a plant-based diet, just not a plant-only one.

As a parent of three children, I want to set a good example for my kids. To teach them to enjoy food, and all the inherent pleasure and social joy it brings. To have them choose healthy foods, including a wide variety of plant foods, because they want to, not because they have to. And to have a healthy relationship with food, and the world around them.

This is an important book at an important time. It delivers something most books about eating better do not: an opportunity for you to not only improve your diet, but also expand your diet. That's easier—and way more delicious—than you think.

YOUR DIET IS NOT A ZERO-SUM GAME. EATING MORE PLANT-BASED FOODS DOES NOT MEAN YOU HAVE TO GIVE UP GOOD SOURCES OF PROTEIN SUCH AS MEAT OR EGGS.

Brian St. Pierre,
M.S., R.D., C.S.C.S.

INTRODUCTION

by Paul Kita

You've done an adventurous thing in picking up this book. Adventurous because you're about to embark on not yet another diet, but a complete transformation in the way you eat. Adventurous because you're about to charge forth into a wild and wonderful world of fruits, vegetables, and grains—including some that you may never have known existed.

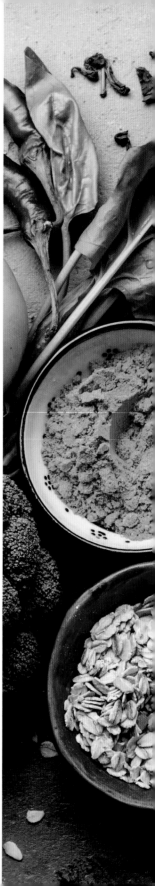

Adventurous because you're about to acquire a powerful new arsenal of nutritious but also incredibly delicious recipes that'll fuel your every day. Adventurous—and also smart—because, as research shows, incorporating more plant-based foods into your meals will propel you to better health, greater energy, and a longer life. And, as a grace note, your plant-based diet may just help the planet live longer, too.

It's understandable if you carry trepidation. This whole "plant-based" thing is new, even to me as the Food & Nutrition Editor of *Men's Health*. In fact, it's new to everyone. Fifteen years ago, if you were to say the words "plant-based" to someone, they might have stared at you, head tilted slightly, and said, "Huh?"

That's because 15 years ago the term didn't really exist. Neither did *Forks Over Knives,* or Impossible Burgers, or fake chicken at KFC. Now it seems that everyone from Mike Tyson to your mother-in-law is eating plant-based, and they're reporting that they've lost weight, dropped their cholesterol levels, and doubled the amount of pep in their step. Some take plant-based eating even further to embrace veganism, where only plant-based products cross their lips.

Recent polling confirms widespread interest in plant-based foods. In fact, a whopping 73 percent of people said they've heard of a "plant-based diet," according to a 2019 survey by the International Food Information Council Foundation. Fifty-one percent of those polled said they would be interested in learning more about a plant-based diet.

UNDERSTANDING PLANT-BASED EATING

According to a 2019 survey by the International Food Information Council Foundation, almost three in four people are familiar with and interested in plant-based diets, yet they aren't quite sure exactly what that means. From that same study, here's how people defined a plant-based diet:

▶ **32%** Vegan diet that avoids all animal products, including dairy and eggs.

▶ **30%** A diet that emphasizes minimally processed foods derived from plants and limits the consumption of animal products.

▶ **20%** A vegetarian (read: no meat, no seafood) diet.

▶ **8%** A diet that limits animal products and encourages eating as many fruits and vegetables as possible.

To clear up this confusion, we worked with experts to define what it means to eat a plant-based diet. Here are the three main principles.

▶ Consume no more than three ounces of meat daily.

▶ Aim to consume at least 25 grams of protein with each meal.

▶ Eat a diet of abundance with a variety of plant-based foods during meals.

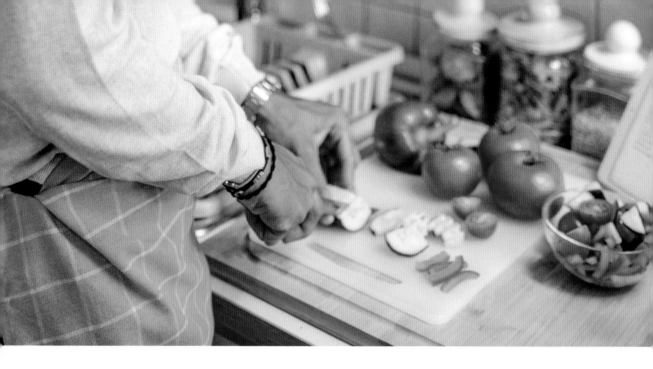

And to complicate all this, neither the USDA nor the FDA currently has a definition for the term "plant-based." In a way, it's similar to the word "natural," in that whoever (or whatever company) can use the term as they see fit and not in accordance with any strict federal guidelines.

And, honestly, the same goes for the medical and research community. In interviewing numerous nutrition, fitness, and sustainability experts for this book, every one of them had different answers to our question: "How would you define a plant-based diet?"

So *Men's Health* built its own definition based on current scientific research and the smartest minds in nutrition, sustainability, and plant-based eating. Follow this plan and you'll add muscle, defend against disease, maintain a healthy weight, and have a ton of energy.

The best part: The *Men's Health* approach to plant-based eating is easy. There's no calorie counting. There's no macro obsession. There's no "ketosis." There's no nonsense.

A Plant-Based Diet Is a Challenge, but an Exciting One

The recipes within this book will include some foods you've never heard of before. Do not wither under intimidation. Track down these products in the grocery store or online, if needed. Take the time required to prep them in your kitchen (don't worry, you'll get the hang of it). Then try them and enjoy them and savor them.

But you also have to level with yourself: You will face challenges. Yes, you will need to make sure that you're consuming enough protein, iron, vitamin B12—which helps your cells function properly—and heart-healthy omega-3 fatty acids. You'll learn how to do this soon—fear not.

You might scour the supermarket for kohlrabi only to discover that it does not carry kohlrabi. You may spend 30 minutes preparing green lentils only to find out that you don't really love green lentils. You may really *really* crave pepperoni pizza. It's okay. Unlike other diets, there's no guilt here. Skip the kohlrabi. Try red lentils. Have a slice (or, heck, two!) of pepperoni pizza. Just keep trying new plant-based foods.

"When a diet is rigid or highly structured, people on those diets are more likely to gain back the weight they lose, report feeling less happy, and are at a greater risk of disordered eating," says Eric Helms, Ph.D., C.S.C.S. "There's no such thing as a bad food—only a bad diet."

A Plant-Based Diet Is Really (Really) Good for You

If you can overcome these challenges, you'll completely overhaul your health. This is largely due to one potent nutrient: fiber. Yawn, right? But fiber is an unsung superhero within the world of healthy eating. Yes, fiber helps you poop, but it also offers so much more than regularity. Fiber fills you up during a meal (what dietitians call "satisfaction"), which can help you eat less at breakfast, lunch, and dinner. Fiber also helps you feel fuller longer after a meal (what dietitians call "satiety"), which can help you eat less between breakfast, lunch, and dinner.

Plus: "Fruits and vegetables also tend to have a very high water content," says Helms. Water, beyond its hydration powers, can also help you feel satisfied simply by taking up space in your stomach. "An entire plate of broccoli is only 30 calories, but it's incredibly filling," he says. That's fiber and water at work. Compare that to a plate of refined pasta, which is much higher in calories and lower in H2O. That pasta can fill you up, Helms says, but not before

THE MEN'S HEALTH PLANT-BASED DIET IS A DIET OF ABUNDANCE

Do not think for a second that a plant-based diet is boring. You do not have to eat tofu if you don't want to you. You do not have to eat beans if you hate beans. You also do not have to subsist upon fake-meat products. You can still eat whatever you want whenever you want. The best approach to eating more plants centers on inclusion.

"Diversity is key," says Chris Vogliano, Ph.D.(c), R.D., a nutrition and sustainability researcher. "It's still a new field, but more research is coming out indicating that our microbiome is stronger and richer if we're eating a more diverse diet." And the healthier your microbiome, science shows, the healthier you are.

Current research finds that a wide and varied diet of healthful foods offers the best benefit for your overall well-being. Which means that you shouldn't have to decide between a beef burger and a black bean burger—it's a diet that includes both beef burgers and black bean burgers. And chickpea burgers, and lentil burgers, and, sure, plant-based "meat" burgers, and other things that aren't burgers, like salmon, tempeh, arugula, barley, apples, oysters, flaxseeds, milk, peanuts, kale, and so much more.

you've taken in more of it than you probably should.

Worry not, carb-loading athletes. A plant-based diet, through nutrient-dense carbohydrates, can still provide a powerful source of energy for short-burst and endurance exercise. Just ask any athlete who has had success training and competing on a regimen powered by plants.

Yet another benefit of a plant-based diet: Fruits and vegetables are strong allies in the fight against disease. Plant-based eating leans hard on nutrient-rich foods. Research shows that dark leafy greens will not only fill you up with fiber, but also deliver payloads of cancer-fighting antioxidants. Nuts and seeds—from peanuts to pistachios to chia—all contain heart-healthy fats. Fermented foods such as tempeh are great for your gut health.

In fact, a 2019 study published in *The Journal of Nutrition* found that vegans tend to live longer than non-vegans. This was not due to an absence of meat, the researchers found, but rather the inclusion of antioxidant-rich and anti-inflammatory foods.

And numerous reports from the last few years also suggest that eating more plants requires farmers to use less land, less water, and less pollution to produce food. Because you might be living a little longer on this planet due to a plant-based diet, you might also want the planet to live a little longer, too.

A Plant-Based Diet Isn't (Always a) Vegan or Vegetarian Diet

A plant-based diet does not mean a diet devoid of all animal products. "A plant-based diet should be an inclusionary diet of plants rather than an exclusionary diet of animal products," says Helms.

Coming from Helms, this is a definitive statement. He's a natural bodybuilder. He's a prolific nutrition and exercise researcher. And he's been on a plant-based diet, as he defines one, for the last 10 years. Unfortunately, Helms says, a battleground has intensified between people who eat meat and people

"A PLANT-BASED DIET SHOULD BE AN INCLUSIONARY DIET OF PLANTS RATHER THAN AN EXCLUSIONARY DIET OF ANIMAL PRODUCTS."
— Eric Helms, Ph.D., C.S.C.S.

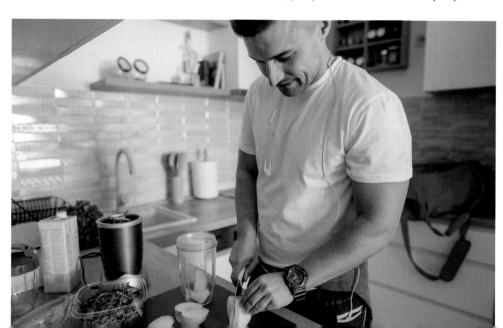

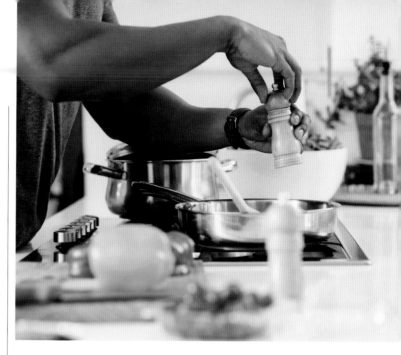

who do not want anyone to eat meat—people who have dug in their heels and emboldened their bases with claims that eating more plants is further evidence that eating no meat is better for you. This is not true.

"From a nutrition science perspective, it's eating more plants that is associated with positive health," Helms says. "Even keto researchers still find a way to keep a high vegetable intake in the diet," referencing the high-fat, high-protein, bacon-approving ketogenic diet.

David Katz, M.D., the founding director of the Yale-Griffin Prevention Research Center, uses the term "plant-predominant." Abby Langer, R.D., a Toronto-based nutrition expert, says that "plant-forward" offers more clarity. Brian St. Pierre, Ph.D., R.D., C.S.C.S., the director of nutrition at Precision Nutrition, a company with clients who include the Carolina Panthers and Houston Rockets, spells it out this way: "The term plant-based usually encourages lots of whole, minimally processed plant foods, such as vegetables, fruits, whole grains, beans, and legumes, as well as nuts and seeds."

None of the experts who informed this book say that you must stop eating animal products to improve your diet. If you want to, go ahead. But it's not essential to better health.

A Plant-Based Diet Isn't a Diet in the Traditional Sense of the Word

You do not have to count calories when you go plant-based. You do not have to manage your macros or, more frustrating, maintain ketosis. You do not have to count points or follow "no-no" lists of banned foods or ingredients, or go through some brutal 30-day "onboarding" or "detox" process.

In fact, going plant-based is all about doing more of one thing: eating fruits, vegetables, legumes, grains, nuts, and seeds. And, in an interesting and counterintuitive way, by doing this one thing, the rest of what you eat—and how you approach eating altogether—balances out. By giving priority to the produce on your plate, you're naturally crowding out the meat from taking up more than its fair share of space.

Plant-based eating grants you the permission to consume more of something instead of focusing on eating less of everything. If you've been a frequent diet dabbler, acknowledge that feeling that should now be arising within you. That feeling is freedom.

Or, as Ryan Andrews, R.D., C.S.C.S., author of *A Guide to Plant-Based Eating*, puts it: "There's not one crash diet that's perfect for everyone forever." In other words, the only diet that will work for you is a diet that works *with* you.

How to Eat Plant-Based in Just Five Steps

1 Put Meat in the Backseat

Andrews urges that you should strive for no more than three ounces of meat daily. Most Americans eat more than that in one sitting. So how do you cut back? When you plan your meals, do so without making meat the centerpiece. "You should build your meals around plants," says Langer. "That doesn't mean that plants have to be the only thing on the plate. That just means thinking about plants first." So, instead of having a big bone-in pork chop for dinner, and then tacking on a side salad, try building a big salad with mixed greens, chickpeas, and then some thinly sliced pork tenderloin on top. Vogliano calls this "using meat as a condiment." Or, if you're making a big batch of chili, halve the amount of ground beef you usually add and double up on the beans. You'll still enjoy the flavors of your food, yet this way of eating encourages you to make plants a priority.

2 But Don't Forget About Protein

With each meal, aim to consume at least 25 grams of protein. This is the minimum amount you need to keep your muscles strong and your stomach full. Protein helps build and maintain strength and mass, and it also helps fill you up. When you reduce the amount of meat you're eating, you need to swap in a high-protein plant food. This is why you're adding chickpeas to the salad in the example in Step 1 (or the delicious Beefy Salad on page 129). Or more beans to the hypothetical chili. Some plant foods that are high in protein: soybeans (and tofu and soy milk),

quinoa, chickpeas, lentils, any kind of nut, peas, any kind of bean, and seitan. You can use an app (a good one: precisionnutrition.com/nutrition-calculator) to track your nutrient intake, or simply follow the recipes in this book that hit that amount. And remember that you can still eat meat, so any meat in that meal counts toward your 25 grams goal.

3 Aim for Abundance

The more diverse your plant-based diet, the better you'll feel—both physically and mentally. St. Pierre suggests that 75 percent of your plate should be made up of plant-based foods. Katz recommends 80 percent of your daily calories come from plants. Expert opinions on the ideal balance of plants to meat may differ, but they all acknowledge that eating *more* plants is a great place to start. If you eat only about one serving of fruit daily, make it a goal to eat two. If you never eat a vegetable for breakfast, try mixing in a handful of spinach to your scrambled eggs (or ask the diner short-order cook to do it).

Plant-based eating also doesn't mean eating the same thing every day. That's boring, and boring diets never work. If you haven't tried snow peas, pick some up at the grocery store and toss them into a stir-fry. Build your salads with a variety of lettuces: romaine, chicory, watercress, arugula, pea shoots, and whatever else looks intriguing. If you ate pork tenderloin early in the week, make sure you're also mixing things up with omega-3-rich fish or B12 rich lamb later in the week. Your goals should include eating more plant-based foods during meals, but also a greater variety of foods overall. Gradually ramp up the plants you eat until you feel good about how many you're eating, or, as Andrews puts it, you find your "minimal effective dose of animal proteins." That's how much animal protein you need to still enjoy it, yet basing the rest of your diet on plants.

4 Go Easy Now

There's no need to go whole-hog on plant-based eating right away. In fact, this isn't a great idea, says Helms. "Any time a diet requires restraint, a willpower clock starts," he says. Remember that there's nothing on the *Men's Health* plant-based diet that you can't have. Andrews says that an easy way to eat more fruit is to have a piece after dinner for dessert in place of your usual ice cream. But if you want ice cream one night, enjoy ice cream. If you eat meat for dinner every night of the week, try building one meatless meal into the rotation weekly—and then maybe two, or even three. Ease yourself into plant-based eating. Small goals, achieved over a long period of time, often lead to big changes. Big goals, achieved over a short period of time, often lead to diet-induced insanity.

5 Enjoy

What you're doing while you eat might be as important as what you're eating. Research shows that eating while distracted interrupts brain-to-stomach satiation signals, making it harder to monitor your food intake. So when you eat, actually *eat*. Grab a seat. Focus on your meal. Don't check your e-mail or hit streaming. Pay attention to your plate. Chew. Savor.

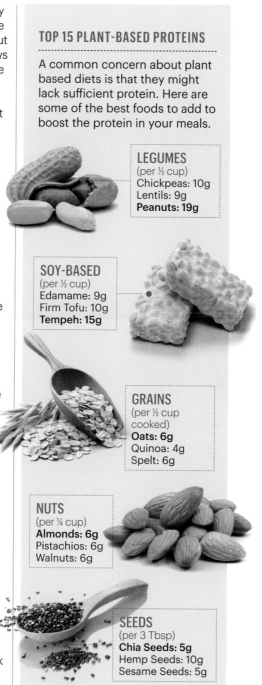

TOP 15 PLANT-BASED PROTEINS

A common concern about plant based diets is that they might lack sufficient protein. Here are some of the best foods to add to boost the protein in your meals.

LEGUMES
(per ½ cup)
Chickpeas: 10g
Lentils: 9g
Peanuts: 19g

SOY-BASED
(per ½ cup)
Edamame: 9g
Firm Tofu: 10g
Tempeh: 15g

GRAINS
(per ½ cup cooked)
Oats: 6g
Quinoa: 4g
Spelt: 6g

NUTS
(per ¼ cup)
Almonds: 6g
Pistachios: 6g
Walnuts: 6g

SEEDS
(per 3 Tbsp)
Chia Seeds: 5g
Hemp Seeds: 10g
Sesame Seeds: 5g

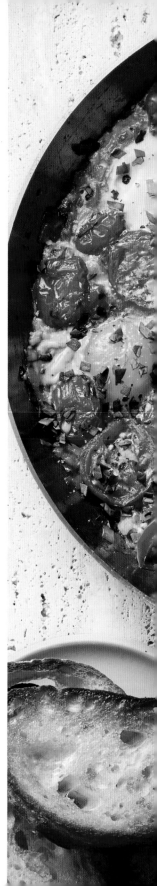

Breakfast

Your first meal of the day can go one of two ways. You could either dial it in (a soggy bowl of sugary cereal, a greasy bag of fast-food, egg-and-mystery-meat sandwiches) or you could spend a little extra time to throw together a breakfast that forms a solid foundation for whatever you're doing that day. When you're going plant-based, breakfast can seem tricky. But with the recipes in this section, you'll find yourself equipped to build meals with staying power and satisfaction—two things cereal boxes and fast-food joints never provide.

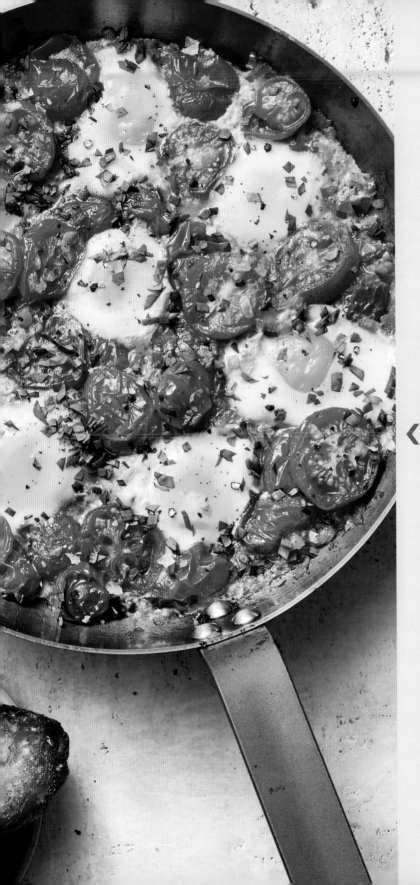

THE RECIPES

Egg Scramble with Sweet Potatoes

SERVES 1

WHAT YOU'LL NEED:

8 OZ DICED SWEET POTATO

½ CUP CHOPPED ONION

2 TSP CHOPPED FRESH ROSEMARY

COOKING SPRAY

4 LARGE EGGS

4 LARGE EGG WHITES

2 TBSP CHOPPED FRESH CHIVES

1. Preheat your oven to 425°F. On a baking sheet, toss the sweet potato, onion, rosemary, ¼ each teaspoon salt and pepper. Lightly coat vegetables with cooking spray then roast until tender, about 20 minutes.

2. Meanwhile, in a small bowl, whisk together the eggs and egg whites, and season with a pinch each of salt and pepper. Coat a large skillet with cooking spray then heat over medium. Add eggs and cook, stirring frequently, until scrambled, 3 to 4 minutes. Sprinkle eggs, potato, and onion with chives.

PER SERVING: *571 calories, 44 g protein, 52 g carbohydrates (9 g fiber), 20 g fat*

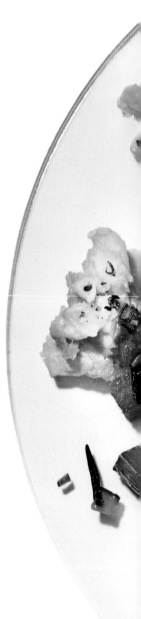

SWEET!

There are many different types of types of sweet potatoes. The flesh can be white, cream-color, golden, and even purple. The most common is the bright orange and very tasty "Covington" variety. A single sweet potato contains 400 percent of the daily recommended amount of vitamin A, which helps keep your eyes and immune system healthy.

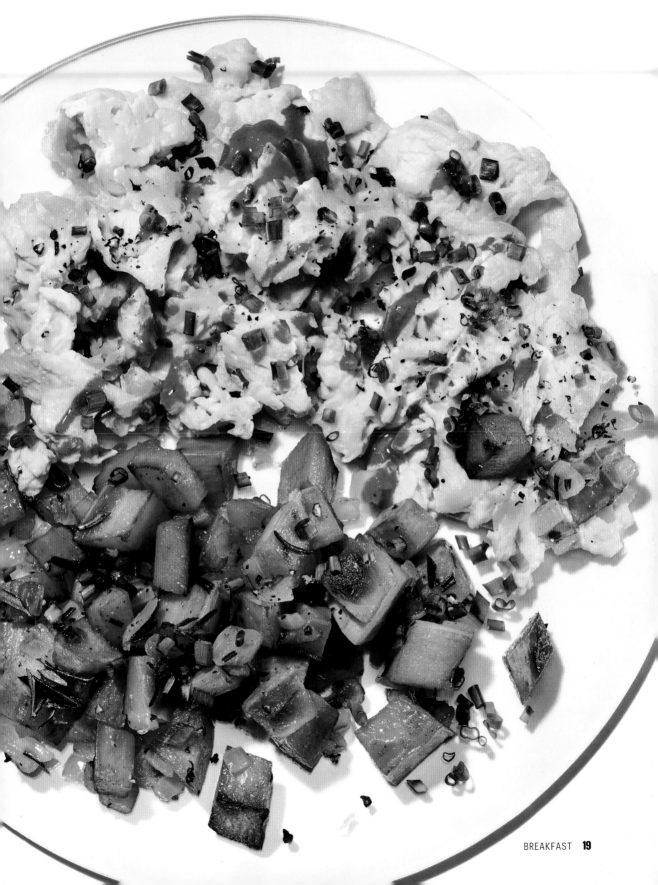

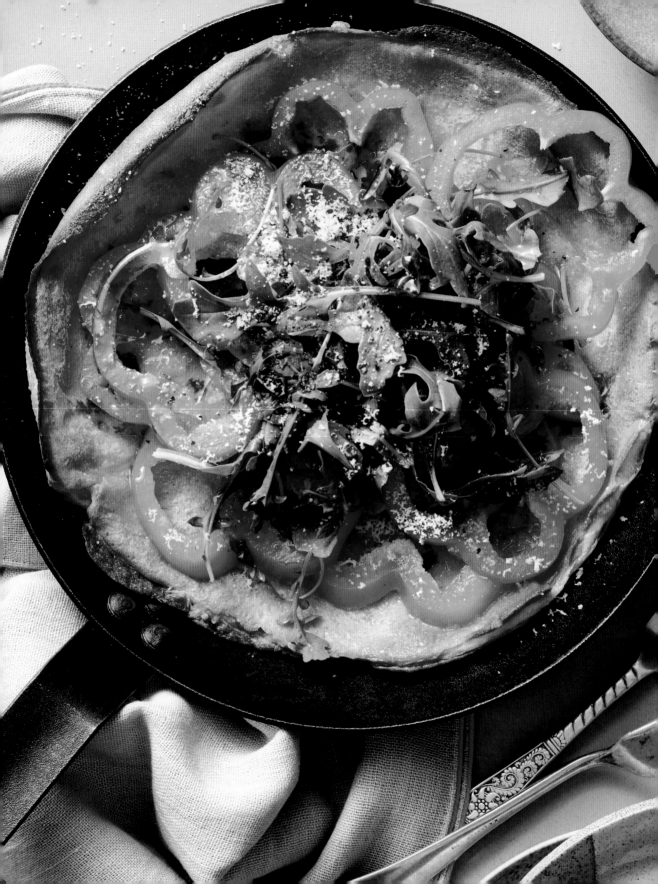

Savory Dutch Baby

SERVES 2

WHAT YOU'LL NEED:

- ⅔ CUP MILK, ROOM TEMPERATURE
- 3 LARGE EGGS, ROOM TEMPERATURE
- ½ CUP + 1 TBSP ALL-PURPOSE FLOUR
- 1 TBSP UNSALTED BUTTER
- 2 CUPS BABY ARUGULA
- 1 ORANGE BELL PEPPER, SLICED CROSSWISE
- 2 TSP BALSAMIC VINEGAR
- 2 TBSP GRATED PARMESAN

1. Position a large cast-iron or oven-safe skillet on the middle rack of your oven and preheat to 425°F.

2. In a blender, combine the milk, eggs, flour, and ½ teaspoon sea salt, and blend until smooth, about 10 seconds.

3. Using oven mitts, carefully remove the skillet from the oven, add butter, and swirl to coat. Pour in batter and bake until puffed and golden brown around edges, 15 to 20 minutes.

4. Meanwhile, in a bowl combine arugula, bell pepper, and vinegar; season with a pinch of salt to taste.

5. Top Dutch Baby with salad then sprinkle Parmesan and season with pepper to taste.

PER SERVING: *385 calories, 19 g protein, 37 g carbohydrates (3 g fiber), 18 g fat*

⫸ PROTEIN BOOST

Top each serving of this beauty with 2 ounces smoked salmon or 2 slices crispy bacon.

POWER MOVE

This Dutch Baby is a savory riff on a sweet German pfannkuchen (also known as Bismarck or Dutch puff). Plus, this recipe has more eggs than flour, so it's heartier. If you're worried that it looks too complicated (oh no, *baking*), all you really have to do is blend together a bunch of ingredients, pour that mixture into a pan, and bake till puffed.

Turmeric Tofu Scramble

SERVES 1

WHAT YOU'LL NEED:

- 1 PORTOBELLO MUSHROOM
- 3 OR 4 CHERRY TOMATOES
- 1 TBSP OLIVE OIL, PLUS MORE FOR BRUSHING
- ½ (14 OZ) BLOCK FIRM TOFU
- 2 TBSP NUTRITIONAL YEAST
- ¼ TSP GROUND TURMERIC
- PINCH GARLIC POWDER
- ½ AVOCADO, THINLY SLICED

1. Preheat your oven to 400°F. Place the mushroom and tomatoes on a baking sheet, then brush with oil, season with salt and pepper, and roast until tender, about 10 minutes.

2. Meanwhile, in a medium bowl, combine the tofu, nutritional yeast, turmeric, garlic powder, and a pinch of salt. Use a fork to crumble it into bite-size pieces. In a large skillet over medium, heat 1 tablespoon oil. Add the tofu and cook, stirring occasionally, until heated through, 3 to 4 minutes.

3. Serve the tofu scramble with the mushroom, tomatoes, and avocado.

PER SERVING: *471 calories, 27 g protein, 21 g carbohydrates (10 g fiber), 33 g fat*

THE MEATIEST MUSHROOM

Portobello mushrooms have an earthy taste and satisfyingly meaty texture, which is why they're often grilled and swapped in for beef burgers. When choosing mushrooms, look for specimens that are firm and dry with no slimy, shriveled, or wet spots. Always remove the stems. Their woody texture is not so great to eat. You can keep the gills on, but if you're adding portobello into, say, a stir-fry, remove them by scraping them with a tip of a spoon. That way the gills won't turn the rest of your meal an unappetizing black color.

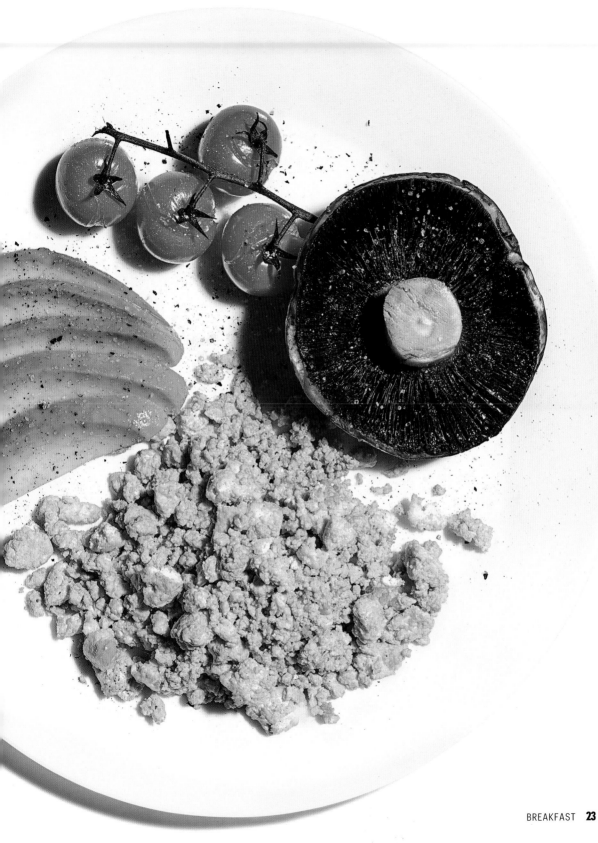

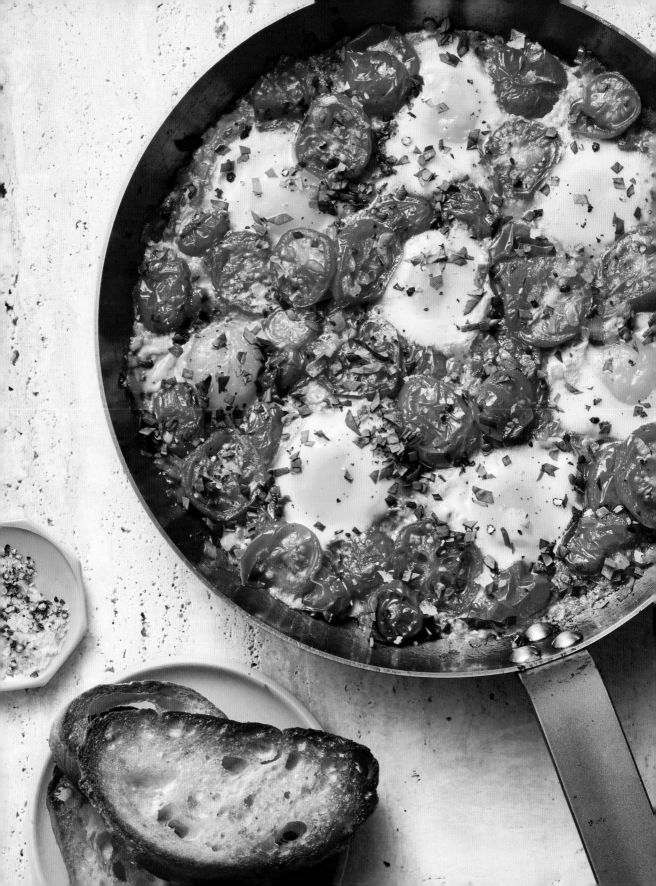

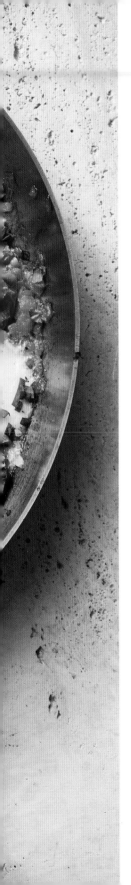

Best-Ever Shakshuka

SERVES 2

WHAT YOU'LL NEED:

2 TBSP OLIVE OIL

1 YELLOW ONION, FINELY CHOPPED

1 GARLIC CLOVE, FINELY CHOPPED

1 TSP GROUND CUMIN

1 LB TOMATOES, HALVED IF LARGE

8 LARGE EGGS

¼ CUP BABY SPINACH, FINELY CHOPPED

SOURDOUGH TOAST OR MULTIGRAIN TOAST, FOR SERVING (OPTIONAL)

1. Preheat your oven to 400°F. In a large oven-safe skillet over medium, heat the oil. Add onion and cook until golden brown and tender, about 8 minutes. Stir in garlic, cumin, ½ teaspoon each salt and pepper and cook 1 minute. Stir in tomatoes.

2. Transfer the skillet to the oven and roast 10 minutes. Carefully remove skillet from the oven. Stir, then make eight small indentations in tomato-onion mixture. Carefully crack one egg into each indentation. Return skillet to the oven.

3. Bake eggs to desired doneness, 7 to 8 minutes for slightly runny yolks. Sprinkle shakshuka with spinach and, if desired, serve with sourdough toast.

PER SERVING: *470 calories, 28 g protein, 16 g carbohydrates (4 g fiber), 34 g fat*

UPGRADE IT

You won't find a better bang for your buck in terms of flavor and ease of prep than this hearty breakfast dish (it's also great for dinner). If you feel like experimenting, stir in a big pinch of smoked paprika or crushed red pepper flakes for an added punch, cooked chickpeas or lentils for a protein boost, or a splash of coconut milk for a creamy component.

Eggs Benedict Florentine with Salmon

SERVES 1

WHAT YOU'LL NEED:

- ½ CUP SPINACH
- 1 LARGE EGG
- 1 EGG YOLK
- 1½ TSP LEMON JUICE
- PINCH OF CAYENNE
- 2 OZ BUTTER, MELTED
- SPLIT ENGLISH MUFFIN HALF, TOASTED
- 3 OZ BAKED SMOKED SALMON, FLAKED

1. Heat a large skillet over medium-low. Add the spinach and a pinch of salt. Cover and cook, stirring occasionally, until wilted, about 5 minutes. Transfer to a paper towel-lined bowl and cover to keep warm.

2. For the poached egg, bring 3 to 4 inches of water to a boil in a wide saucepan. Add ½ teaspoon salt and reduce heat. Carefully crack the egg into the water and simmer over low until white is set, 4 to 7 minutes. Remove the egg with a slotted spoon and drain on a paper towel.

3. For the hollandaise sauce, in a blender, add egg yolk, lemon juice, a big pinch of salt, and the cayenne. With the blender running, gradually add butter and blend until emulsified.

4. Add the spinach to the muffin then top with salmon, the poached egg, and hollandaise.

PER SERVING: *722 calories, 29 g protein, 15 g carbohydrates (1 g fiber), 61 g fat*

BE LIKE POPEYE

Eaten raw or cooked, spinach is a superfood packed with vitamins, minerals, fiber, and antioxidants. It's loaded with heart-healthy vitamins A and C, vitamin K for bone health, magnesium for metabolism, and potassium, which can help balance the effects of sodium on the body.

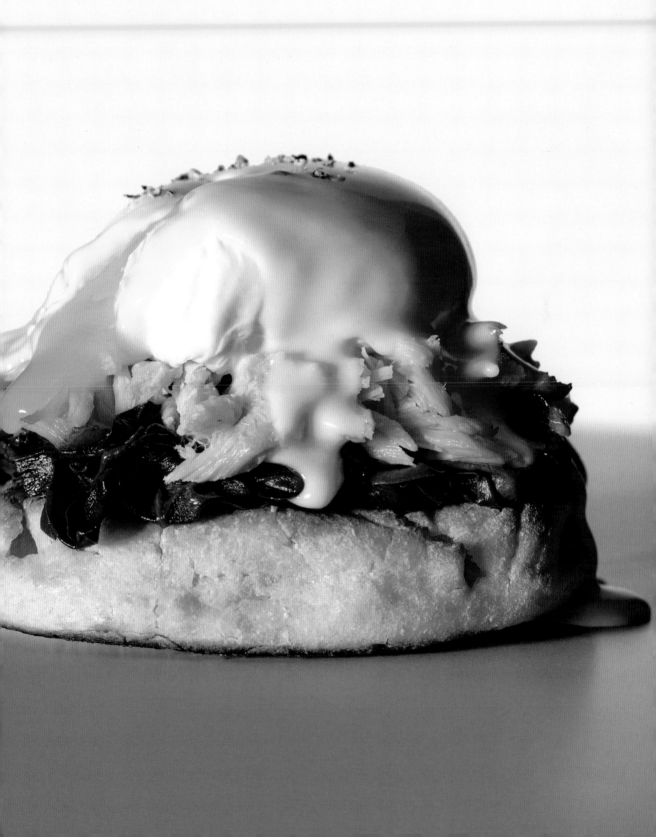

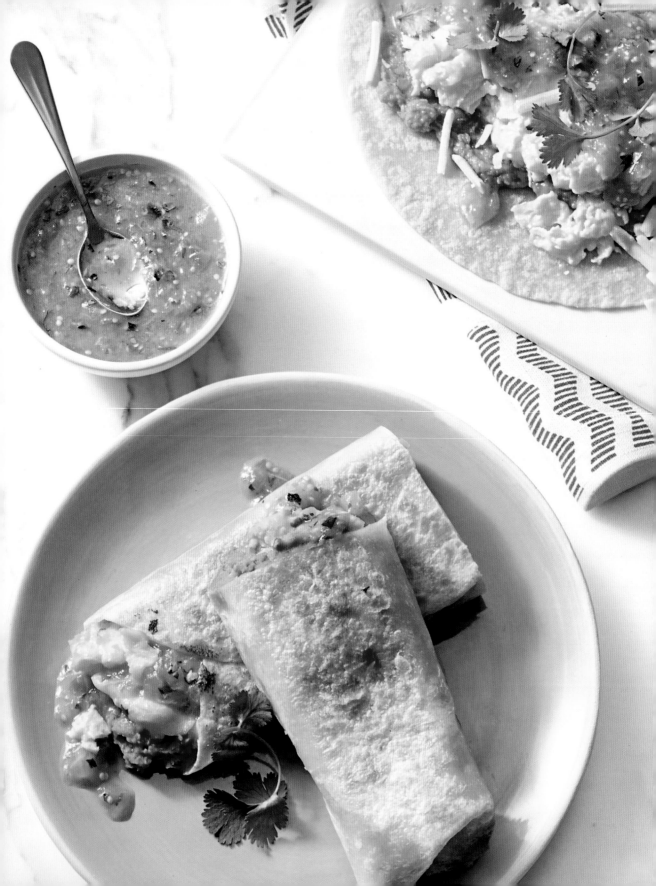

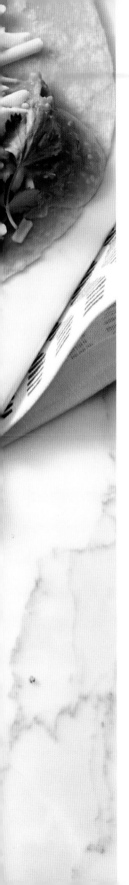

Breakfast Burritos

SERVES 4

WHAT YOU'LL NEED:

½ LB TOMATILLOS, HUSKED, RINSED, AND HALVED

1 JALAPEÑO, HALVED AND SEEDED

½ SMALL ONION, CUT INTO WEDGES

JUICE FROM 1 LIME

⅓ CUP PACKED FRESH CILANTRO

6 LARGE EGGS

1 TSP OLIVE OIL

1 CUP SHREDDED PEPPER JACK OR CHEDDAR CHEESE

1 CUP FAT-FREE REFRIED BEANS

4 LARGE TORTILLAS

FRESH CILANTRO

1. Arrange oven rack 6 inches from broiler; preheat broiler.

2. For the salsa, place tomatillos and jalapeño, cut sides down, on a foil-lined baking sheet along with onion and broil until blistered, 10 to 12 minutes. Let cool, then transfer to a food processor. Add lime juice, cilantro, and ¼ teaspoon kosher salt and pulse to combine (salsa should be slightly chunky).

3. In a small bowl, beat eggs with 1 tablespoon water and ¼ teaspoon kosher salt. In a large nonstick skillet, heat the oil over medium. Add eggs and cook, stirring frequently, until scrambled, 3 to 4 minutes. Fold in ½ cup cheese.

4. To assemble burritos, spread ¼ cup refried beans on each tortilla, then divide eggs and remaining cheese on top. Spoon 2 tablespoons salsa over each burrito and sprinkle with the additional cilantro. Roll, folding sides over filling and then rolling from bottom up. If desired, crisp both sides of burrito in the nonstick skillet over medium. Serve with remaining salsa.

PER SERVING: *485 calories, 25 g protein, 49 g carbohydrates (4 g fiber), 22 g fat*

WRAP, FREEZE, AND ROLL

Freeze foil-wrapped burritos up to three weeks. To reheat, remove foil and microwave until heated through, thee to five minutes.

Mexican Breakfast Nachos

SERVES 4

WHAT YOU'LL NEED:

- 6 LARGE EGGS
- ½ TBSP CANOLA OIL
- 5 OZ TORTILLA CHIPS
- 1 CUP SHREDDED MONTEREY JACK CHEESE
- ¼ CUP PICKLED JALAPEÑO SLICES
- 1 AVOCADO, THINLY SLICED
- 1 CUP PICO DE GALLO
- 2 TBSP FRESH CILANTRO, CHOPPED
- SOUR CREAM AND LIME WEDGES, FOR SERVING (OPTIONAL)

1. In a small bowl, beat eggs with ¼ teaspoon salt. In an oven-safe 12-inch nonstick skillet, heat the canola oil over medium. Add eggs and cook, stirring frequently, until scrambled, 3 to 4 minutes. Transfer to a bowl and set aside. Wipe skillet clean.

2. Preheat broiler. Spread half the chips in the same skillet. Sprinkle with half the cheese. Top with remaining chips and cheese, then eggs and jalapeño. Broil until cheese is melted and chips begin to brown, 1 to 2 minutes.

3. Remove from oven; top with avocado, pico de gallo, and cilantro. If desired, serve with sour cream and lime wedges.

PER SERVING: *495 calories, 19 g protein, 36 g carbohydrates (6 g fiber), 32 g fat*

PROTEIN BOOST

Toss 2 ounces leftover chicken or beef or one cup black beans on this hearty skillet breakfast to hit 25 g protein.

GET ON TOP OF YOUR GAME

These loaded nachos also make for a hearty appetizer before the big game. Swap out the egg for black beans, pinto beans, or plant-based meat crumbles. You can also change up the toppings to suit your craving. And the best part? They're ready in just 20 minutes.

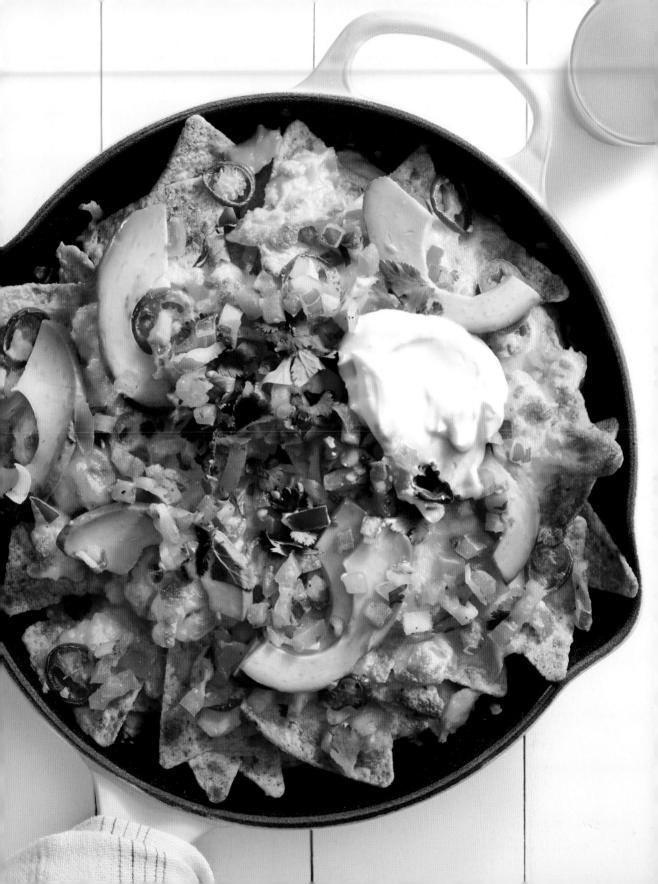

Mocha Muscle Oatmeal >

SERVES 2

WHAT YOU'LL NEED:

⅔ CUP STEEL-CUT OATS

¼ TO ½ CUP MILK

1 SCOOP (35 G) CHOCOLATE PROTEIN POWDER

1 TSP INSTANT COFFEE

¼ TSP CARDAMOM

1 CUP SLICED STRAWBERRIES

¼ CUP CHOPPED ALMONDS

MILK, FOR SERVING (OPTIONAL)

1. In a medium saucepan over medium heat, add the oats, a pinch of salt, and 1¾ cups water. Bring to a simmer, then remove the pan from the heat. Cover, refrigerate, and let the oats soak overnight.

2. In the morning, stir in milk to your liking, protein powder, instant coffee, and cardamom.

3. Heat the oatmeal over medium-low for 5 minutes, stirring a couple times, until heated through. Transfer to bowls, top with strawberries and almonds, and serve with a splash of milk, if desired.

PER SERVING: *448 calories, 25 g protein, 55 g carbohydrates (12 g fiber), 15 g fat*

PB Oatmeal

SERVES 3

WHAT YOU'LL NEED:

½ CUP STEEL-CUT OATS

2 TBSP PEANUT BUTTER

1 SCOOP (35 G) CHOCOLATE PROTEIN POWDER

½ SLICED BANANA

1 TBSP RAISINS

1 TBSP CHOPPED WALNUTS

1. In a small saucepan over medium heat, add the oats, a pinch of salt, and 1⅓ cups water. Bring to a simmer, then remove the pan from the heat. Stir in peanut butter. Cover, refrigerate, and let the oats soak overnight.

2. In the morning, stir in the protein powder. Heat the oatmeal over medium-low for 5 minutes, stirring a couple times, until heated through. Transfer to bowls, then top with banana, raisins, and walnuts.

PER SERVING: *740 calories, 42 g protein, 84 g carbohydrates (13 g fiber), 28 g fat*

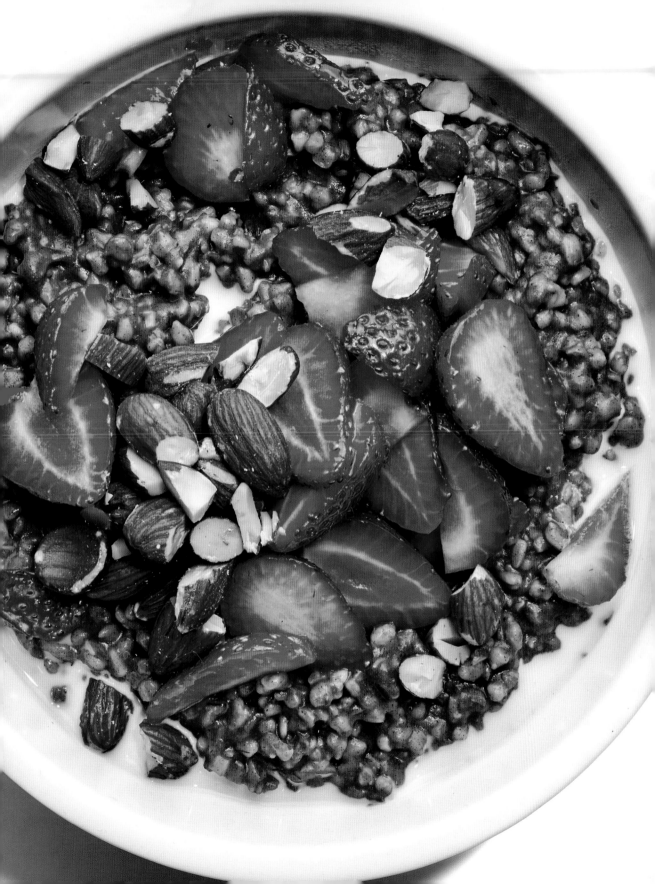

"Candied" Yams Oatmeal

SERVES 2

WHAT YOU'LL NEED:

⅔ CUP STEEL-CUT OATS

¼ TO ½ CUP MILK

½ CUP MASHED SWEET POTATO

1 SCOOP (35G) VANILLA PROTEIN POWDER

¼ TSP NUTMEG

2 TBSP ALMOND BUTTER

2 TSP MAPLE SYRUP

MILK, FOR SERVING (OPTIONAL)

1. In a medium saucepan over medium, add the oats, a pinch of salt, and 1¾ cups water. Bring to a simmer, then remove pan from the heat. Cover, refrigerate, and let the oats soak overnight.

2. In the morning, stir in milk to your liking, sweet potato, protein powder, and nutmeg.

3. Heat the oatmeal over medium-low for 5 minutes, stirring a couple times, until heated through. Transfer to bowls, then top with almond butter and maple syrup, and serve with a splash of milk, if desired.

PER SERVING: *503 calories, 26 g protein, 67 g carbohydrates (12 g fiber), 16 g fat*

BOOST FIBER WITH OATS

If you need to eat more fiber, oatmeal is a wise place to start. One cup of cooked oatmeal contains four grams of fiber, a nutrient that promotes heart and gut health and helps improve blood sugar levels. Oatmeal contains the extra-special soluble fiber called beta-glucan. Because beta-glucan itself isn't digested, it slows food in transit in the intestines, resulting in lower cholesterol, improved blood sugar management, and a well-functioning immune system.

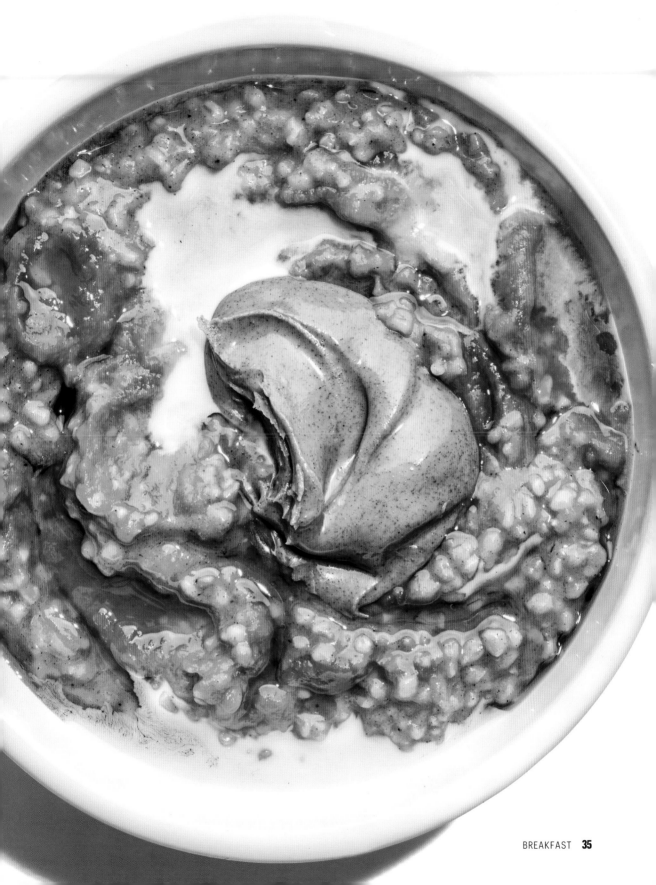

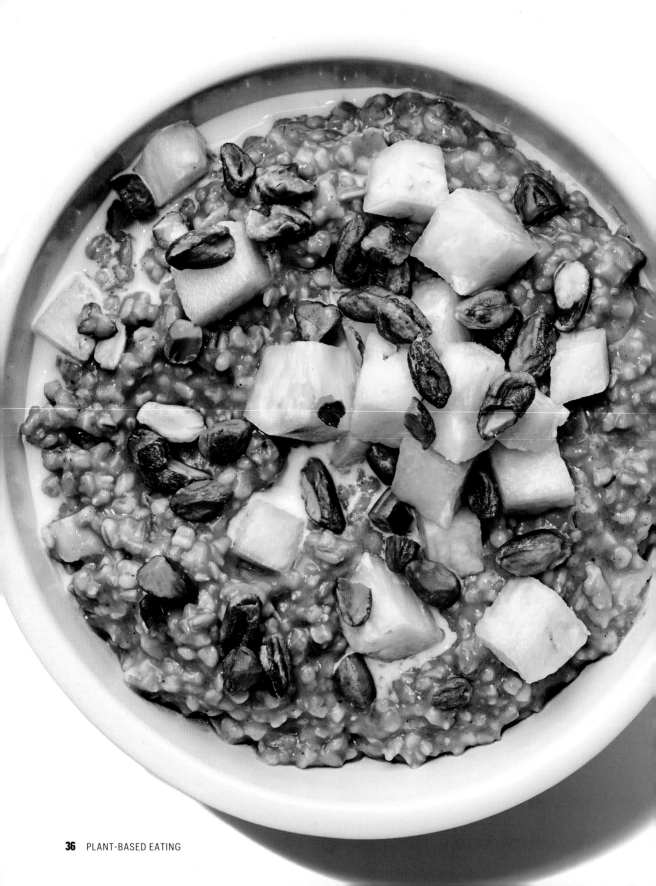

Green Machine Oatmeal

SERVES 2

WHAT YOU'LL NEED:

- ⅔ CUP STEEL-CUT OATS
- ¼ TO ½ CUP MILK
- 1 TSP MATCHA POWDER
- 2 TBSP SHREDDED COCONUT
- ½ TSP GROUND GINGER
- 1 CUP CHOPPED PINEAPPLE
- ¼ CUP CHOPPED PISTACHIOS
- MILK, FOR SERVING (OPTIONAL)

1. In a medium saucepan over medium heat, combine the oats, a pinch of salt, and 1¾ cups water. Bring the water to a simmer, then remove the pan from the heat. Cover, refrigerate, and let the oats soak overnight.

2. In the morning, stir in milk to your liking, matcha powder, shredded coconut, and ginger.

3. Heat the oatmeal over medium-low for 5 minutes, stirring a couple times, until heated through. Transfer to bowls, then top with pineapple and pistachios, and serve with a splash of milk, if desired.

PER SERVING: *430 calories, 16 g protein, 58 g carbohydrates (10 g fiber), 16 g fat*

||⊢→ **PROTEIN BOOST**

Add ½ a scoop of vanilla protein powder for a high protein breakfast.

MATCHA'S GOTCHA

Vibrant green matcha comes from the same plant that all green, black, and oolong teas come from: *Camellia sinensis*. The powder is made by grinding the whole leaf, which is rich in antioxidants called polyphenols. So when you eat matcha powder, you're eating a good dose of disease-fighting antioxidants. Tastes good going down, too.

Berry Bowl >

SERVES 3

WHAT YOU'LL NEED:

- 1½ CUPS PLAIN 2% GREEK YOGURT
- ¼ CUP BLUEBERRIES
- ¼ CUP RASPBERRIES
- ¼ CUP SLICED STRAWBERRIES
- ¼ CUP BLACKBERRIES
- ¼ CUP UNSALTED DRY-ROASTED SHELLED PISTACHIOS
- ¼ CUP UNSWEETENED COCONUT FLAKES

Spoon yogurt into bowls, then top with berries, pistachios, and coconut.

PER SERVING: *621 calories, 37 g protein, 43 g carbohydrates (11 g fiber), 36 g fat*

Savory Grits

SERVES 1

WHAT YOU'LL NEED:

- 1 TBSP OLIVE OIL
- 2 TBSP FINELY CHOPPED SHALLOT
- ½ CUP LOW-SODIUM CHICKEN BROTH
- 1 PACKET (1 OZ) INSTANT GRITS
- 2 TBSP NUTRITIONAL YEAST FLAKES
- 2 LARGE EGGS
- 1 RADISH, THINLY SLICED
- ½ AVOCADO, THINLY SLICED

1. In a saucepan over medium, heat oil. Add the shallot and cook until soft, about 2 minutes. Add the broth and bring to a boil.

2. Pour the grits into a bowl, then add the nutritional yeast and hot broth, and stir until the grits have thickened.

3. For the poached egg, bring 3 to 4 inches of water to a boil in a wide saucepan. Add ½ teaspoon salt and reduce heat. Carefully crack the eggs into the water and simmer over low until white is set, 4 to 7 minutes. Remove the eggs with a slotted spoon and drain on a paper towel.

4. Top the grits with eggs, radish, and avocado, and season with pepper.

PER SERVING: *511 calories, 26 g protein, 39 g carbohydrates (10 g fiber), 31 g fat*

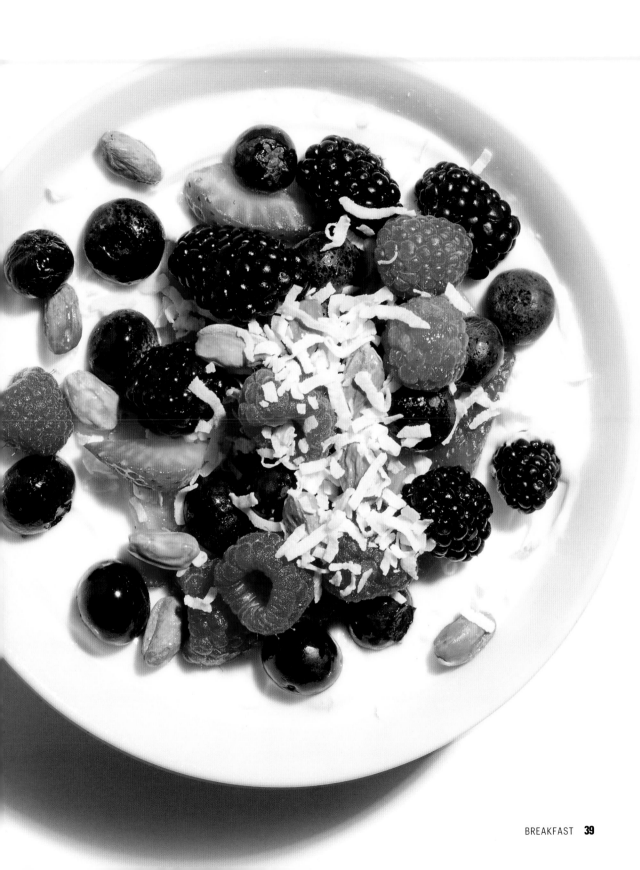

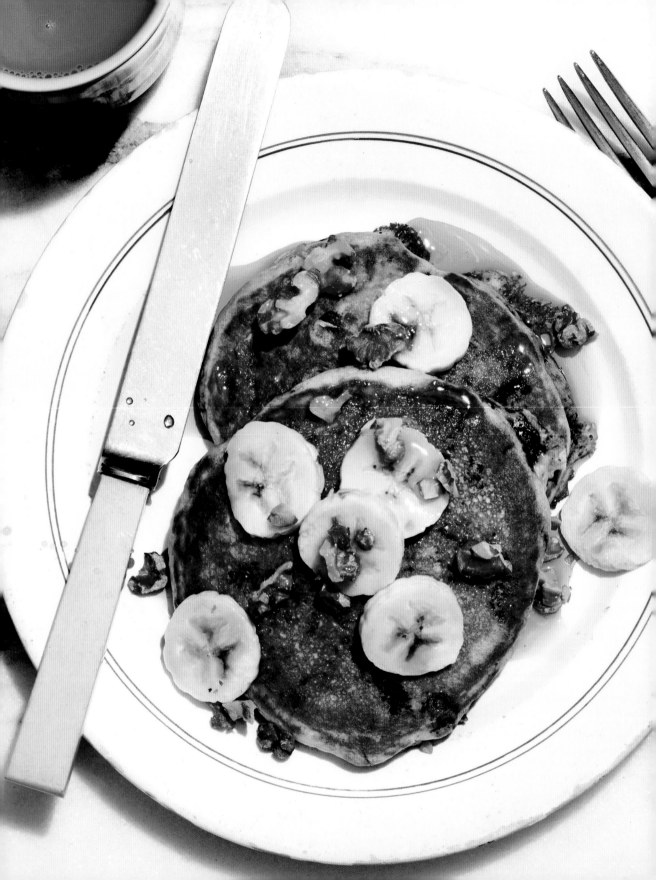

Blueberry-Banana Pancakes

SERVES 2

WHAT YOU'LL NEED:

1 CUP HIGH-PROTEIN PANCAKE AND WAFFLE MIX (SUCH AS KODIAK CAKES)

½ CUP FROZEN BLUEBERRIES

OLIVE OIL, FOR BRUSHING

½ CUP CHOPPED WALNUTS

1 BANANA, SLICED

MAPLE SYRUP, FOR SERVING

1. In a large bowl, whisk together the pancake mix with 1 cup cold water until combined (don't overblend). Stir in the blueberries.

2. Brush a large nonstick skillet with olive oil and heat over medium. Working in batches, add ¼ cup batter per pancake to the pan. Cook until bubbles appear, about 2 minutes. Flip and cook until the undersides are golden brown, about 1 to 2 minutes.

3. Serve immediately with walnuts, banana, and maple syrup, if desired. Makes six 4-inch pancakes.

PER SERVING: *463 calories, 17 g protein, 56 g carbohydrates (9 g fiber), 22 g fat*

⊪→ PROTEIN BOOST

Add a bowl of plain yogurt topped with berries. Choose Greek yogurt for 15 to 20 grams of protein, or regular yogurt for eight to nine grams of protein per serving.

MIX IT UP

Pancakes are super versatile. Switch up the stir-ins and this becomes a whole new recipe. Try fresh or frozen raspberries and chopped almonds; fresh or frozen chopped peaches and pecans; or chopped apples and walnuts. You can use dried fruit, too. Stir in chopped dried apricots and unsweetened coconut flakes or dried cranberries and chopped pistachios.

Bear-Size PB&J ❯

SERVES 1

WHAT YOU'LL NEED:

- 2 HIGH-PROTEIN FREEZER WAFFLES (SUCH AS KODIAK CAKES)
- 2 TBSP CRUNCHY PEANUT BUTTER
- ⅓ CUP MIXED STRAWBERRIES AND BLACKBERRIES, CHOPPED
- 2 TBSP HIGH-PROTEIN GRANOLA

Toast the waffles according to package directions. While still warm, spread the peanut butter over one waffle. Top with the berries, granola, and remaining waffle.

PER SERVING: *682 calories, 27 g protein, 54 g carbohydrates (10 g fiber), 41 g fat*

Super Waffles

SERVES 1

WHAT YOU'LL NEED:

- 2 HIGH-PROTEIN FREEZER WAFFLES (SUCH AS KODIAK CAKES)
- 1 CUP PLAIN YOGURT
- 2 SLICED PEACHES
- 2 TBSP UNSALTED DRY-ROASTED SHELLED PISTACHIOS
- 2 TBSP WHOLE FLAXSEEDS
- FRESH MINT, TORN

Toast the waffles according to package directions. Place waffles on a plate and top with yogurt, peaches, pistachios, flaxseeds, and mint.

PER SERVING: *629 calories, 32 g protein, 85 g carbohydrates (13 g fiber), 23 g fat*

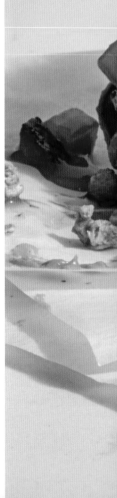

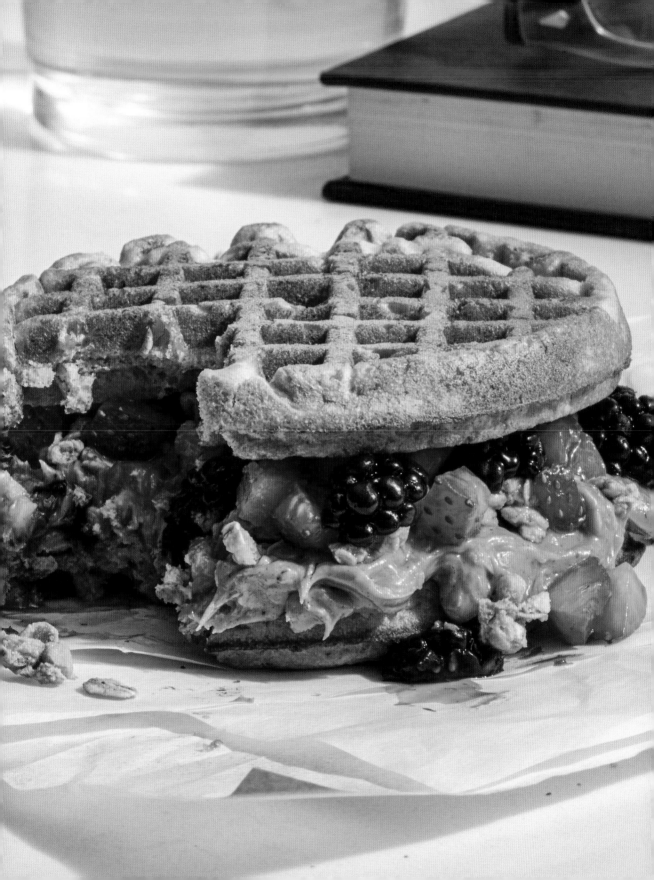

Plant-Based Fitness Fuel

Shakes are a great way to deliver nutrients to your body fast. A well-built shake contains a strong dose of protein, but also healthy fats and fiber. Instead of entrusting the contents of your shake to a smoothie shop, avoid all the sugar and calories and go DIY. These plant-based shakes are a great place to start.

SMOOTHIE AND SHAKE DIY

Protein: Add a scoop of protein powder—whey or plant-based. See page 158 for our picks.

Fat: Measure out a single serving of high-fat additions, like nut butters, flax and chia seeds, or avocados.

Greens: Add a handful of greens, like kale or spinach, to boost antioxidants and fiber and feel full longer.

Fruit: Start with about 1 cup of fruit per smoothie. When using apples, leave the skin on for extra phytonutrients.

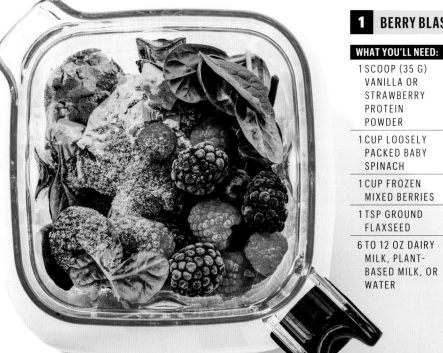

1 BERRY BLAST SUPER SHAKE

WHAT YOU'LL NEED:

1 SCOOP (35 G) VANILLA OR STRAWBERRY PROTEIN POWDER

1 CUP LOOSELY PACKED BABY SPINACH

1 CUP FROZEN MIXED BERRIES

1 TSP GROUND FLAXSEED

6 TO 12 OZ DAIRY MILK, PLANT-BASED MILK, OR WATER

In a blender, combine the protein powder, spinach, berries, and flaxseed. Puree until well combined, then add the liquid until the desired consistency is achieved. Serves 1.

PER SERVING:
290 calories, 31 g protein, 31 g carbohydrates (6 g fiber), 7 g fat

2 CHERRY-BANANA SHAKE

WHAT YOU'LL NEED:

8 OZ UNSWEETENED ALMOND MILK

2 OZ TART CHERRY JUICE

1 BANANA

1 SCOOP (35G) PROTEIN POWDER

1 RAW EGG (SHELL OPTIONAL)

In a blender, combine almond milk, juice, banana, protein powder, and egg. Puree until smooth. Serves 1.

PER SERVING:
366 calories,
32 g protein,
39 g carbohydrates
(4 g fiber), 13 g fat

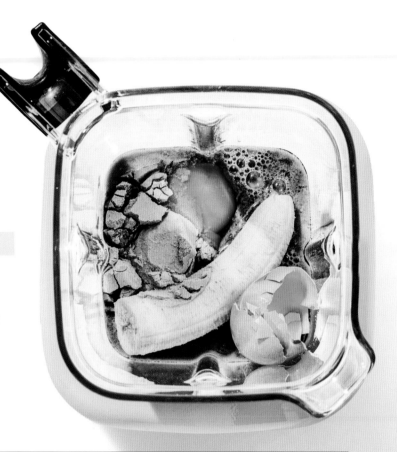

3 CHOCOLATE-BANANA SHAKE

WHAT YOU'LL NEED:

1 SCOOP (35 G) CHOCOLATE PROTEIN POWDER

1 FROZEN BANANA

1 HEAPING TBSP PEANUT BUTTER

8 TO 10 OZ VANILLA UNSWEETENED ALMOND MILK

HANDFUL ICE CUBES

In a blender, combine the protein powder, banana, and peanut butter. Puree until well combined, then add the almond milk and ice until the desired consistency is achieved. Serves 1.

PER SERVING:
445 calories,
26 g protein,
53 g carbohydrates
(6 g fiber), 15 g fat

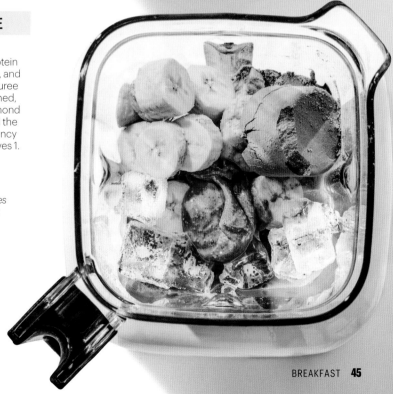

Coconut Raspberry Cashew Shake >

SERVES 1

WHAT YOU'LL NEED:

1⅓ CUPS UNSWEETENED
   COCONUT MILK
   BEVERAGE

1 SCOOP (35G) PROTEIN
   POWDER

½ CUP FROZEN
   RASPBERRIES

1 TBSP CASHEW BUTTER

2 TSP AGAVE SYRUP

In a blender, combine coconut milk beverage, protein powder, raspberries, cashew butter, and agave syrup. Puree until smooth.

PER SERVING: *422 calories, 30 g protein, 44 g carbohydrates (1 g fiber), 15 g fat*

Chocolate-Cherry Super Shake

SERVES 1

WHAT YOU'LL NEED:

2 SCOOPS (70G)
   CHOCOLATE PROTEIN
   POWDER

2 CUPS FRESH OR FROZEN
   SWEET DARK CHERRIES,
   PITS REMOVED

1 CUP FRESH SPINACH

1 TBSP WALNUTS

1 TBSP GROUND FLAXSEED

1 TBSP DARK COCOA
   POWDER

In a blender, combine 12 ounces water, protein powder, cherries, spinach, walnuts, flaxseed, and cocoa powder. Puree until smooth.

PER SERVING: *585 calories, 59 g protein, 38 g carbohydrates (8 g fiber), 22 g fat*

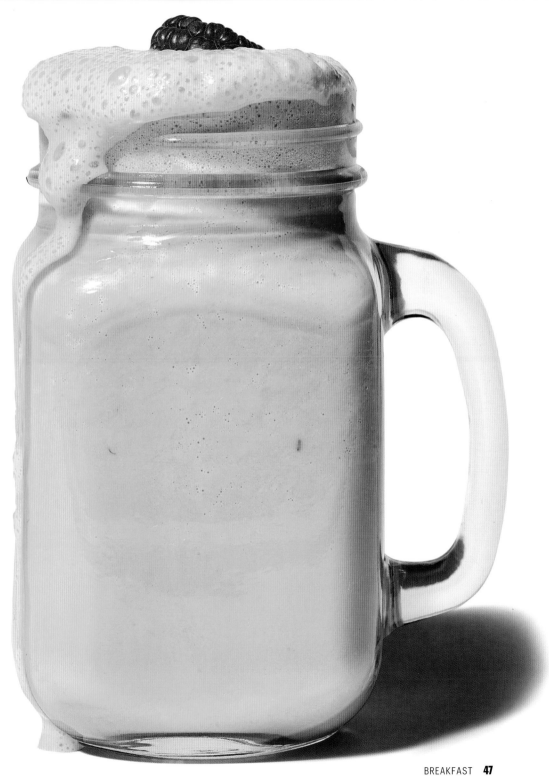

Plant-Based Protein Powders

If you're plant-based curious and looking to build muscle, consuming enough protein—the macronutrient fuel that's necessary for muscular growth—can pose a challenge.

When it comes to protein powder, whey is considered the gold standard for guys who want to build muscle fast. It packs all the amino acids you need for muscle growth and repair, and is also high in leucine, the most important amino acid in the muscle-building process. But whey doesn't work for everyone, and if you're adopting a plant-based diet, you definitely need options.

Can you really build muscle with plant-based protein powder? Turns out the answer is yes—you just have to buy the right kind.

You should opt for a protein powder that mixes different types of plant proteins. This ensures you're consuming all the essential amino acids and a wider range of nutrients.

Most plant-based protein powders come with a few grams of added sugar, and that's by necessity, according to Marie Spano, R.D., C.S.C.S., a sports nutritionist for the Atlanta Hawks. Without it they'd taste like dirt and would be about as hard to mix. Blend protein powder with a few ounces of orange juice to boost the vitamin and nutrient content and offset the "earthy" taste. After all, you'll never reap the benefits of plant-based protein powders if you can't force yourself to drink them.

Here are our picks for the best plant-based protein powders you can buy.

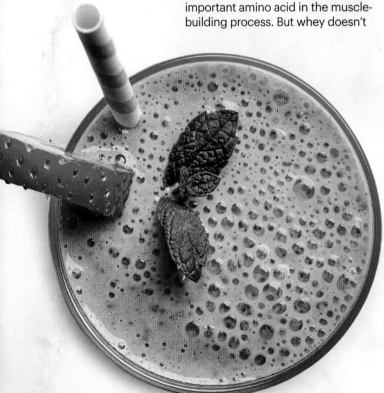

BEST ALL AROUND

Vega Sport Protein Powder, Chocolate Made from a mix of peas, pumpkin, organic sunflower seeds, and alfalfa, one 22-gram scoop of this protein powder contains 30 grams of protein and only 80 calories. Plus, it contains 2.9 grams of leucine—more than you'd find in many whey protein powders.

BEST INGREDIENTS

Garden of Life Meal Replacement, Chocolate Made with proteins from peas, brown rice, amaranth, buckwheat, chia seeds, and more, one 36-gram scoop packs 20 grams of protein, plus a 7-gram dose of fiber.

BEST UNIQUE MIX

Sunwarrior Warrior Blend, Vanilla Made from a blend of Goji berries and pea and hemp proteins, each 25-gram scoop contains 18 grams of protein and about 2.6 grams of muscle-building leucine.

BEST DO-EVERYTHING MIX

Vega One All-In-One Plant-Based Protein Powder, French Vanilla A combination of pea protein, flaxseed, hemp protein, and more, one hefty 41-gram scoop contains 20 grams of protein, 6 grams of fiber, and 1.5 grams of omega-3 fatty acids.

BEST ENHANCED POWDER

Organifi Complete Protein Made from a mix of pea protein, quinoa, pumpkin seeds, coconut, and monk fruit, this protein powder is packed with vitamins from whole foods and digestion soothing enzymes.

BEST GYM BAG OPTION

Garden of Life Organic Protein Powder A totable pouch because you can't throw a tub into your bag. Well, unless you have one of those giant body bags.

BEST LOW-CALORIE

Thorne Research VegaLite Vegan-Friendly Performance Protein Powder, Vanilla This 20 grams-of-protein-per-scoop powder has only 110 calories.

Bowls & Power-Packed Plates

The only people who complain about a plant-based diet being "too hard," are the people who aren't willing to strike out into the unknown when it comes to new flavors. The taste combos in this section may not be what you're used to—but that's exactly the point. Plus, they're easy meals: pastas, stir-fries, sheet-pan feasts. So even if you try one and it's not your thing, no sweat. On to the next one.

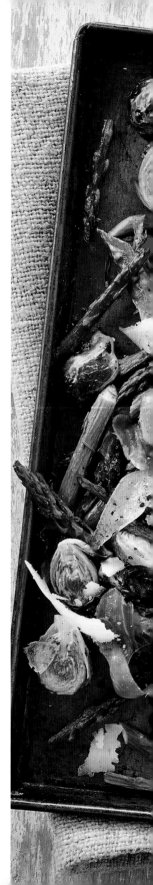

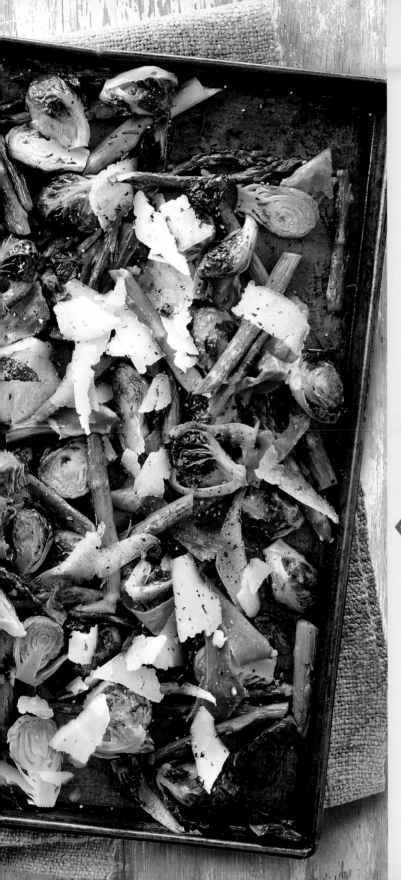

THE RECIPES

Roasted Vegetable Bowl

SERVES 4

WHAT YOU'LL NEED:

CILANTRO-LIME BLACK BEANS

- 1 (15 OZ) CAN BLACK BEANS, RINSED
- ½ TSP GROUND CUMIN
- ¼ CUP CHOPPED FRESH CILANTRO
- JUICE FROM 1 LIME

MAPLE-CHILI SWEET POTATOES

- 2 TBSP OLIVE OIL
- 2 TBSP MAPLE SYRUP
- 1 TSP CHILI POWDER
- ¼ TSP CAYENNE PEPPER
- 2 MEDIUM SWEET POTATOES, CHOPPED INTO ½-INCH CHUNKS

MARINATED MUSHROOMS

- 2 TBSP BALSAMIC VINEGAR
- 2 TBSP OLIVE OIL
- 1 TBSP DIJON MUSTARD
- 1 LB CREMINI MUSHROOMS, HALVED

ROMESCO SAUCE

- 1 CUP ROASTED RED PEPPERS
- ½ CUP PACKED FRESH PARSLEY
- ¼ CUP SALTED ROASTED ALMONDS

PARMESAN PANKO CRUMBS

- 1 TBSP OLIVE OIL
- ½ CUP PANKO
- 2 TBSP FINELY CHOPPED FRESH PARSLEY
- 2 TBSP GRATED PARMESAN

FOR SERVING

- 1 (5 OZ) BAG SPINACH
- ¼ CUP CRUMBLED FETA

1. Prepare the beans. In a small saucepan over medium, heat the black beans, cumin, and ½ teaspoon salt until warm. Add cilantro and lime juice. Set aside.

2. Prepare the potatoes. Preheat your oven to 425°F. In a large bowl, whisk together the oil, syrup, chili powder, cayenne, and ¼ teaspoon salt, then toss with the sweet potatoes. Roast on a rimmed baking sheet until golden brown and tender, stirring halfway through, 35 to 40 minutes.

3. Prepare the mushrooms. Whisk together the vinegar, oil, Dijon, ¼ teaspoon each salt and pepper. Toss with the mushrooms. Roast on another rimmed baking sheet in the same oven until liquid has evaporated, 20 minutes.

4. Prepare the sauce. In a food processor, pulse red peppers, parsley, almonds, and a pinch of salt until almost smooth.

5. Prepare the Parmesan panko crumbs. In a small skillet over medium-low, heat the oil. Add panko, stirring, until golden brown, about 3 minutes. Transfer to a small bowl; add the parsley and Parmesan.

6. In a large bowl, assemble the spinach, beans, potatoes, mushrooms, sauce, crumbs, and crumbled feta.

PER SERVING: *510 calories, 16 g protein, 58 g carbohydrates (14 g fiber), 25 g fat*

⊪⟶ PROTEIN BOOST

Toss 2 ounces leftover sliced steak, chicken, tofu, tempeh, or salmon on each bowl.

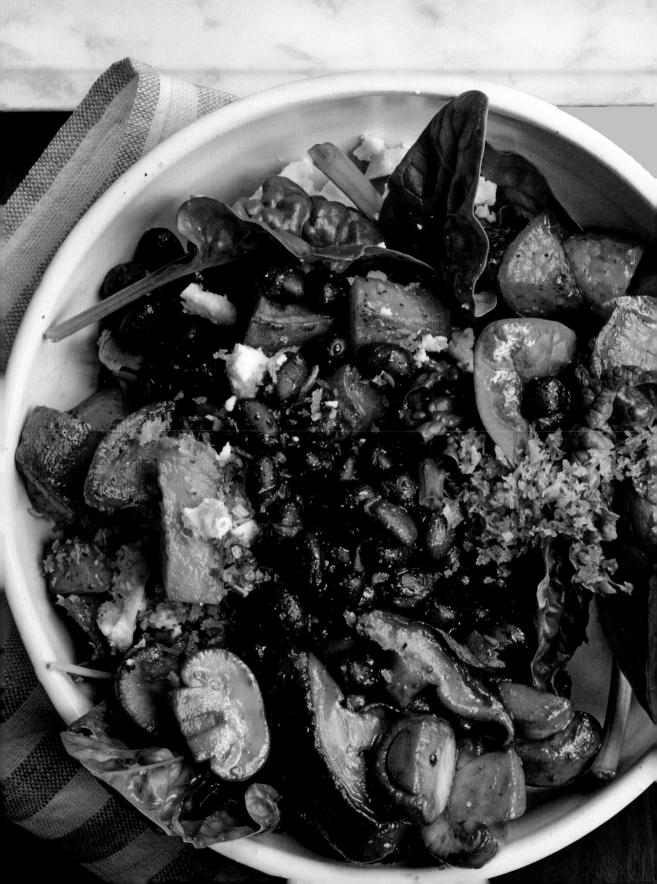

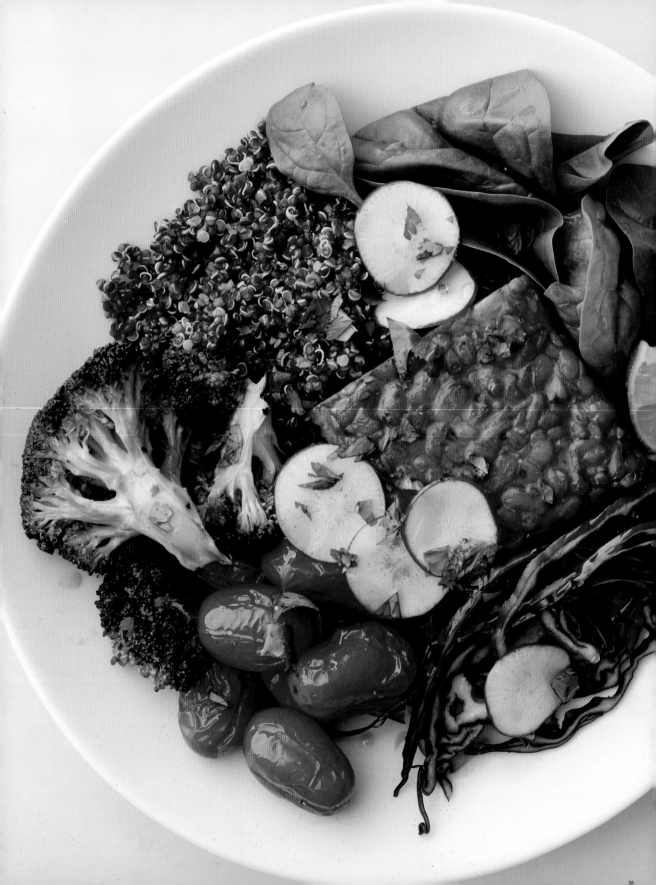

Roasted Vegetables and Tempeh Bowl

SERVES 1

WHAT YOU'LL NEED:

1 (8 OZ) PACKAGE TEMPEH

¼ CUP REDUCED-SODIUM TAMARI

3 TBSP OLIVE OIL

2 TBSP LIME JUICE

6 CLOVES GARLIC, MINCED

1 TBSP GRATED FRESH GINGER

1 CUP BABY SPINACH

½ CUP SHREDDED RED CABBAGE

½ CUP COOKED QUINOA

1 CUP LEFTOVER ROASTED VEGETABLES (SUCH AS ½ CUP EACH GRAPE TOMATOES AND BROCCOLI)

2 TBSP CHOPPED FRESH CILANTRO

¼ TSP TOASTED SESAME OIL

SLICED RADISHES AND LIME WEDGE, FOR SERVING

1. Preheat your oven to 425°F. Cut the tempeh crosswise into 2 pieces and place in a foil-lined baking pan.

2. In a small bowl, whisk together the tamari, olive oil, lime juice, garlic, and ginger. Spoon the tamari mixture over the tempeh and turn to coat the other side. Roast until golden brown, 12 to 15 minutes. Let cool.

3. In a large bowl, combine the spinach, cabbage, quinoa, roasted vegetables, and 1 piece of the tempeh. (Refrigerate remaining tempeh in an airtight container for another use.) Sprinkle with the cilantro and drizzle with sesame oil. Top with sliced radishes and lime.

PER SERVING: *639 calories, 36 g protein, 50 g carbohydrates (9 g fiber), 36 g fat*

MIX IT UP

This meal is versatile: Swap chicken for the tempeh, cooked farro for the quinoa, and kale for the spinach. And lemon juice or even grapefruit juice works just as well as lime.

Tahini-Lemon Quinoa with Shaved Asparagus

SERVES 4

WHAT YOU'LL NEED:

- 1 (19 OZ) CAN CHICKPEAS, RINSED AND DRAINED
- ZEST AND JUICE OF 1 LEMON
- 1¼ CUPS QUINOA
- 10 TBSP TAHINI
- JUICE FROM 2 LIMES
- 1 TBSP HONEY
- 1 CUP PACKED FRESH MINT LEAVES
- 1 LB THICK ASPARAGUS, TRIMMED
- ½ CUP CHOPPED PISTACHIOS

1. In a bowl, combine the chickpeas, lemon zest and juice, and a pinch each of salt and pepper. Let sit 20 minutes then drain.

2. Meanwhile, cook the quinoa according to package directions then season with a pinch of salt.

3. In a blender, puree the tahini, lime juice, honey, mint, ½ cup water, and ¼ teaspoon salt until smooth, adding additional water if needed.

4. With a vegetable peeler, shave the asparagus into ribbons, peeling from the woody end toward the tip.

5. Divide the cooked quinoa, asparagus ribbons, and marinated chickpeas among 4 bowls. Sprinkle with pistachios and drizzle with tahini dressing.

PER SERVING: *657 calories, 25 g protein, 75 g carbohydrates (15 g fiber), 32 g fat*

SHAVE YOUR ASPARAGUS

Cooked and raw asparagus have been used since ancient Greek and Roman times as a natural diuretic. The distinct odor you might notice when you urinate shortly after eating asparagus is from an amino acid, asparagusic, which breaks down into a sulfur-containing compound when digested. Eaten raw in its original spear shape, asparagus can be tough. Shaved into ribbons, it's tender yet crisp.

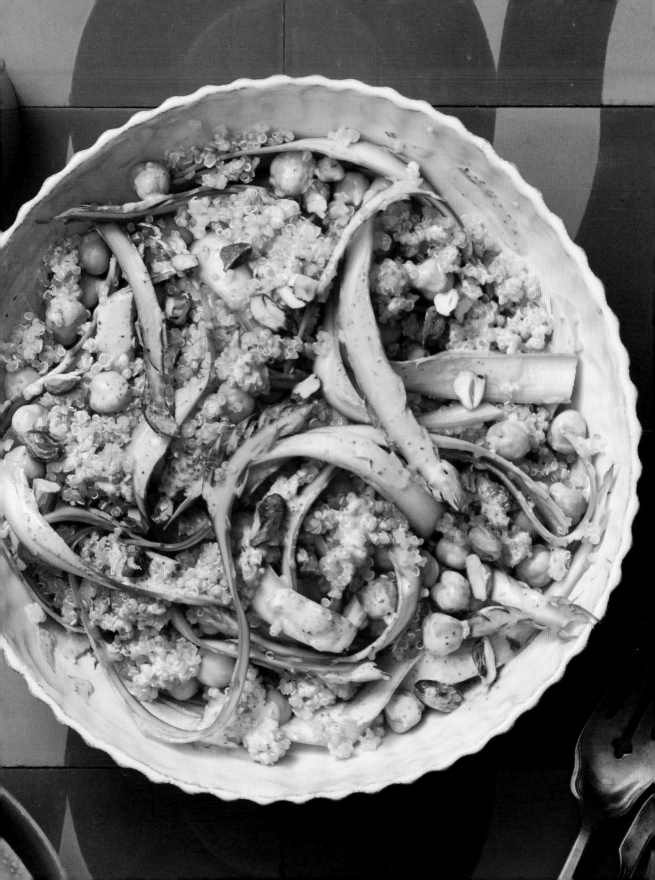

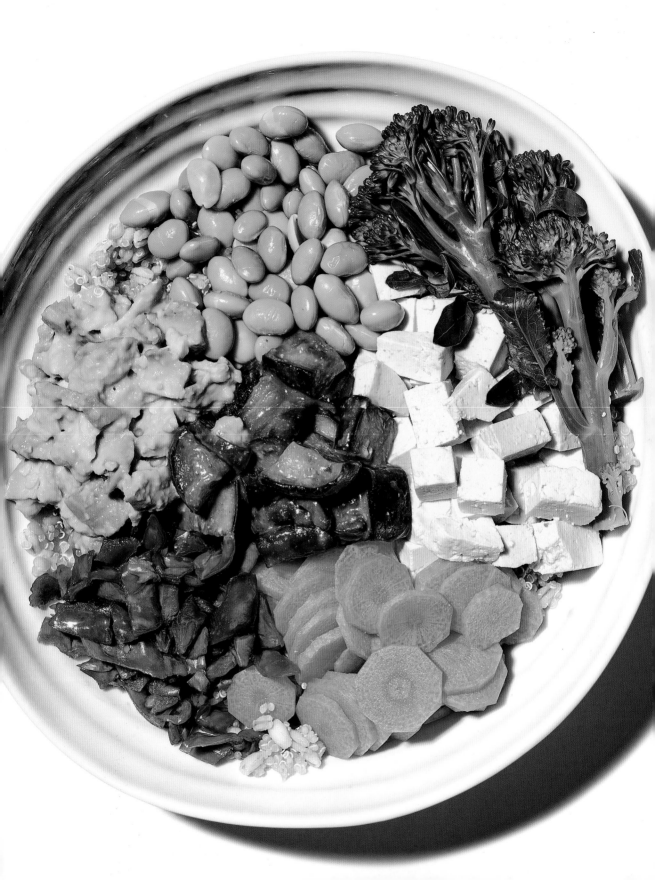

Miso Eggplant Grain Bowl

SERVES 3

WHAT YOU'LL NEED:

- ½ CUP QUINOA, RINSED
- ¼ CUP PEARL BARLEY
- ¼ CUP LENTILS
- 1 TBSP WHITE MISO PASTE
- 2 TSP MIRIN
- 1 TSP SOY SAUCE
- 2 TBSP CANOLA OIL, DIVIDED
- 1 SMALL EGGPLANT, DICED
- 2 CUPS BROCCOLINI
- 2 TBSP SESAME DRESSING
- ½ CUP DICED EXTRA-FIRM TOFU
- ½ CUP FROZEN SHELLED EDAMAME, THAWED
- ½ CUP DICED AVOCADO
- ½ CUP PICKLED RED CABBAGE
- ½ CUP THINLY SLICED CARROT

1. In a medium saucepan, combine the quinoa, barley, lentils, and 1¾ cups water. Bring to a boil, uncovered, and then reduce the heat to low. Cover and simmer until the grains are tender, 15 to 20 minutes.

2. In a small bowl, whisk together the miso, mirin, soy sauce, and 1 teaspoon water. Set aside.

3. In a large skillet over medium, heat 1 tablespoon canola oil. Add the eggplant and cook until browned, turning halfway through cooking, 6 to 8 minutes. Add the reserved sauce and simmer, stirring, until saucelike, 2 minutes. Transfer to a plate.

4. Wipe out the pan, add the remaining 1 tablespoon canola oil, and return it to medium heat. Add the Broccolini and cook until slightly charred and tender, about 3 minutes. Season with a pinch of salt. Transfer to the plate with the eggplant.

5. Toss the grains with the dressing and divide among three bowls. Top with eggplant, Broccolini, tofu, edamame, avocado, cabbage, and carrot.

PER SERVING: *652 calories, 29 g protein, 92 g carbohydrates (23 g fiber), 21 g fat*

EGGPLANT: A MASTER CLASS

This fruit (yes, fruit) does it all. It grills! It roasts! It pan-sears! It purees with oil into a silky dip! Ripe eggplants are at their peak when they feel firm and look shiny, with taut skin. For perfectly browned eggplant with crisp edges and a tender center, make sure to use a well-oiled cooking surface and ensure that the oil is hot before adding the eggplant. (A good visual test: if you see wisps—not plumes—of smoke rising from the pan, it's hot.)

Crispy Chickpea and Kale Bowl

SERVES 4

WHAT YOU'LL NEED

FARRO

⅔ CUP FARRO, RINSED

GARLICKY KALE

2 TBSP OLIVE OIL

2 LARGE GARLIC CLOVES, FINELY CHOPPED

1 LARGE BUNCH KALE, STEMMED AND CHOPPED

TOMATO SALAD

1 PINT CHERRY TOMATOES, HALVED

1 TBSP OLIVE OIL

1 SCALLION, SLICED

CRISPY CHICKPEAS

1 (15 OZ) CAN CHICKPEAS

1 TBSP OLIVE OIL

FOR SERVING

1 AVOCADO, CHOPPED

1. Prepare the farro. In a medium saucepan, bring 1½ cups water to a boil. Add ½ teaspoon salt and farro and return to a boil, then reduce heat to medium-high. Cook, uncovered, until soft, about 30 minutes. Drain.

2. Prepare the kale. In a large skillet over medium, heat the oil. Add the garlic and cook until golden brown, 1 minute. Add the kale, a handful at a time, tossing until wilted before adding more. Season with ¼ teaspoon each salt and pepper and cook until just tender, 3 to 4 minutes.

3. Prepare the tomato salad. In a large bowl, toss the cherry tomatoes, oil, scallions, and a pinch each of salt and pepper.

4. Prepare the chickpeas. Preheat your oven to 425°F. Rinse and drain chickpeas; pat dry with paper towels, discarding any loose skins. Place chickpeas on a rimmed baking sheet; toss with olive oil, ½ teaspoon each salt and pepper. Roast, shaking pan occasionally, until crisp, about 40 minutes.

5. Divide the farro, kale, tomato salad, chickpeas, and avocado among four bowls.

PER SERVING: *427 calories, 13 g protein, 48 g carbohydrates (12 g fiber), 23 g fat*

⫘→ **PROTEIN BOOST**

Grill a plant-based burger or sausage to serve alongside this bowl of good.

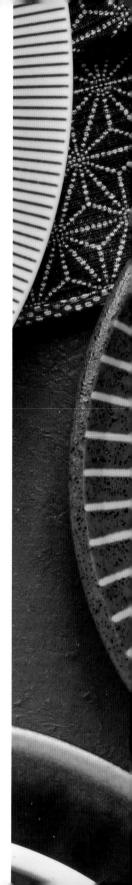

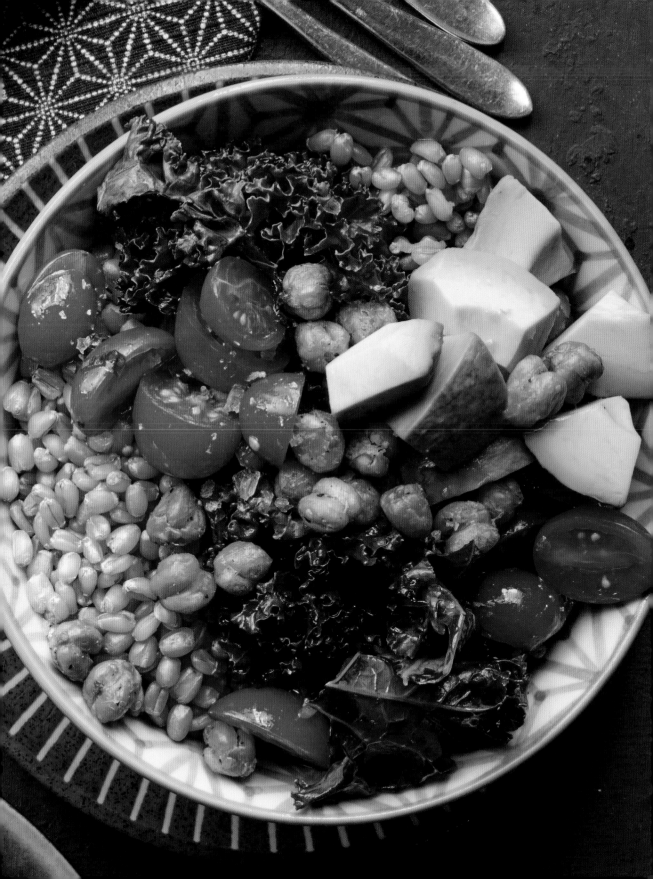

Almond Broccoli Rabe Pasta with Shrimp

SERVES 1

WHAT YOU'LL NEED:

- 1 TBSP OLIVE OIL
- 4 LARGE PEELED AND DEVEINED SHRIMP
- 2 GARLIC CLOVES, MINCED
- ¼ CUP UNSALTED ALMONDS, ROUGHLY CHOPPED
- 1 LB BROCCOLI RABE, CHOPPED
- 2 OZ WHOLE-WHEAT SPAGHETTI, COOKED
- 1 TBSP GRATED PARMESAN

1. In a skillet, heat the olive oil over medium. Add the shrimp, garlic, almonds, and broccoli rabe and cook until the shrimp are pink, about 2 minutes.

2. Toss the shrimp mixture with the cooked spaghetti and sprinkle with Parmesan.

PER SERVING: *708 calories, 38 g protein, 70 g carbohydrates (13 g fiber), 35 g fat*

THEY'RE BUDS, BUT NOT FAMILY

Broccoli and broccoli rabe are both known for their green stalks and clusters of flowery buds—and they can be used interchangeably in most recipes. But it's a common misconception that they're related. Broccoli is a cruciferous vegetable in the *Brassiscacea* family (same as cabbage and kale, among others). Broccoli rabe—which has thinner stalks and a slightly bitter taste—is in the turnip family.

Cauliflower Poke Bowl

SERVES 4

WHAT YOU'LL NEED:

2 TBSP LOW-SODIUM SOY SAUCE

2 TSP RICE VINEGAR

1 TSP SRIRACHA

1 TSP SESAME OIL

1 TSP HONEY

1 SCALLION, THINLY SLICED

2 LARGE CAULIFLOWER HEADS, CUT INTO ½-INCH CUBES

2 CUPS COOKED SUSHI RICE

TOPPINGS

CUBED AVOCADO, CARROTS, RADISH SLICES, CRUSHED MACADAMIA NUTS, TORN NORI, AND SESAME SEEDS

1. In a bowl, whisk the soy sauce, 1 tablespoon water, rice vinegar, sriracha, sesame oil, honey, and scallion.

2. In a pot of boiling salted water, cook the cauliflower cubes just until tender, about 2 minutes. Drain and transfer to the bowl with the sauce and toss to coat the cauliflower. Refrigerate for 1 hour or overnight.

3. To serve, divide sushi rice and cauliflower among four bowls. Top with the avocado, carrots, radish, macadamia nuts, torn nori, and sesame seeds.

PER SERVING: *370 calories, 13 g protein, 55 g carbohydrates (12 g fiber), 14 g fat*

⫸ PROTEIN BOOST

Make a traditional poke bowl with 8 ounces sushi-grade fish like raw yellowfin (ahi) tuna, salmon, or snapper. Want to keep it vegan? Add 14 ounces cubed tofu.

CAULIFLOWER POWER

Poke (psst ... it's pronounced POH-keh) means "to slice or cut" in the Hawaiian language, and most often refers to chunks of raw, marinated fish tossed over rice and topped with vegetables and umami-packed sauce. This plant-based version swaps the usual tuna for fibrous cauliflower. Plus, just one cup of raw cauliflower delivers about 75 percent of the RDA of your daily vitamin C recommendation.

Vegetable Lo Mein

SERVES 4

WHAT YOU'LL NEED:

- 1 (8 OZ) PACKAGE WHOLE-GRAIN SPAGHETTI
- 1 (10 OZ) PACKAGE FROZEN CHOPPED BROCCOLI
- 1½ CUP FROZEN SHELLED EDAMAME
- 2 CUPS SHREDDED CARROTS
- 1 (10 OZ) PACKAGE BABY SPINACH
- 2 TBSP TOASTED SESAME OIL
- 1 LARGE ONION, THINLY SLICED
- 2 TSP GRATED FRESH GINGER
- ¼ CUP LOW-SODIUM SOY SAUCE
- 2 TBSP BALSAMIC VINEGAR
- 1 CUP CRUMBLED FIRM TOFU

1. In a large pot, cook the spaghetti according to package instructions. Just before draining, add the broccoli, edamame, carrots, and spinach. Drain and set aside.

2. In the same pot over medium-high, heat sesame oil. Add the onion and cook for 5 minutes. Add the ginger, soy sauce, and vinegar and cook for 1 minute.

3. Stir in the tofu and cook 1 minute. Add the noodle mixture and cook, tossing, for 2 minutes or until heated through.

PER SERVING: *460 calories, 25 g protein, 63 g carbohydrates (15 g fiber), 15 g fat*

FORGET LOW CARB

All carbohydrates are not created equal. High-quality, nutrient-dense carbohydrates (like the whole-grain spaghetti in this recipe) offer filling fiber. Compared to processed carbohydrates, like refined pasta and bread, whole-grain carbohydrates are nutritional powerhouses. Enjoy them.

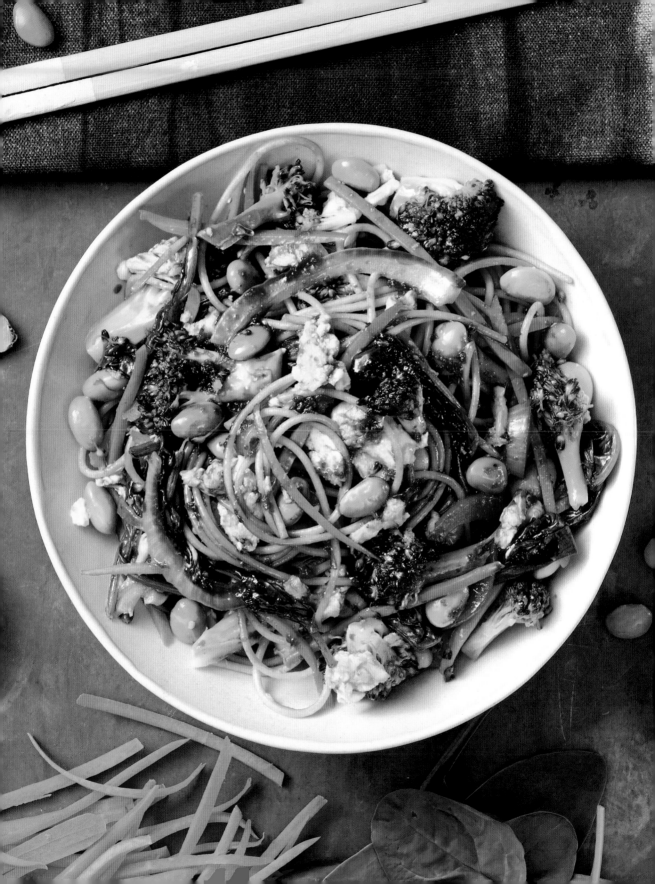

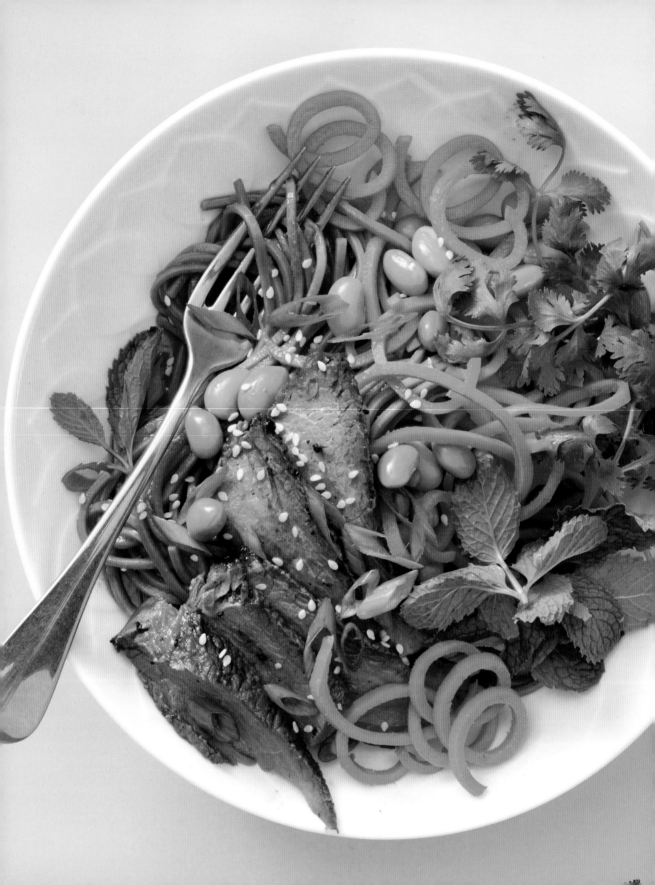

Asian Steak Noodle Bowl

SERVES 4

WHAT YOU'LL NEED:

- 8 OZ BUCKWHEAT SOBA NOODLES
- 8 OZ SIRLOIN STEAK
- 1 TBSP OLIVE OIL
- 2 TBSP RICE VINEGAR
- 2 TSP SESAME OIL
- 1 TSP CHILI PASTE
- 1 CUP SPIRALIZED CARROTS
- 1½ CUPS FROZEN SHELLED EDAMAME, THAWED
- ½ CUP FRESH MINT
- ½ CUP FRESH CILANTRO
- TOASTED SESAME SEEDS AND SLICED SCALLIONS, FOR SERVING

1. In large pot, cook soba noodles according to package directions. Drain then rinse with cold water, and refrigerate while cooking the steak.

2. Season steak with salt and pepper. In a cast-iron skillet over medium-high, heat olive oil. Add steak and cook to desired doneness, 5 to 7 minutes per side for medium. Let rest 5 minutes before slicing.

3. In a large bowl, whisk together vinegar, sesame oil, chili paste, and ½ teaspoon salt. Add soba noodles and carrots and toss to coat. Stir in edamame, mint, and cilantro.

4. Divide noodle mixture among four bowls, then top with sliced steak and sprinkle with sesame seeds and scallions.

PER SERVING: *438 calories, 25 g protein, 51 g carbohydrates (7 g fiber), 16 g fat*

SOY NUTRITIOUS

Japanese restaurants serve shell-on edamame as a hot appetizer. Dunked in soy sauce, and popped out of their pods with your teeth, it's a fun way to start a meal. But edamame, which is actually a type of soy bean, is actually really good for you. It's a great source of plant protein and has a decent amount of fiber. You can buy them without their shells on (check the freezer section) to save you on some prep.

Spicy Stuffed Squash

SERVES 3

WHAT YOU'LL NEED:

1 TSP + 1 TBSP OLIVE OIL

1 LEEK, WHITE AND LIGHT-GREEN PARTS ONLY, FINELY CHOPPED, RINSED WELL

3 CELERY RIBS, CHOPPED

12 OZ MIXED MUSHROOMS, ROUGHLY CHOPPED

1 CUP CANNED CHICKPEAS, RINSED AND DRAINED

1 TBSP SOY SAUCE

¾ CUP CHOPPED WALNUTS

¼ CUP TOMATO PUREE

1 TSP SMOKED PAPRIKA

½ TSP CAYENNE PEPPER

1 (2½ LB) BUTTERNUT SQUASH, SLICED LENGTHWISE, SEEDED

1. Preheat your oven to 350°F. In a large pan over medium, heat 1 teaspoon oil. Add the leek and celery and cook, stirring occasionally, until softened, 2 to 3 minutes. Add the mushrooms, chickpeas, and soy sauce. Cook, stirring occasionally, until the mushrooms release their moisture, about 5 minutes.

2. Add the walnuts, tomato puree, paprika, and cayenne. Simmer until well incorporated, about 5 minutes. Season with salt and pepper. Remove the skillet from the heat.

3. Place the squash on a baking sheet and rub with 1 tablespoon oil; season with salt and pepper. Fill the squash with the mushroom mixture. Roast the stuffed squash in the oven until tender, 30 to 40 minutes.

PER SERVING: *527 calories, 17 g protein, 67 g carbohydrates (15 g fiber), 27 g fat*

⫸ PROTEIN BOOST

Add a high-protein side such as precooked lentils with a squeeze of lemon.

ON THE SIDE

Pair this sweet-and-spicy stuffed squash with a salad of iron- and calcium-rich dark leafy greens. Wash, dry, and coarsely chop a mess of collard greens or kale (any kind). Drizzle some olive oil over the leaves, and massage with your fingers for a couple of minutes to tenderize them. Drizzle with Lemon-Tahini Dressing on page 89.

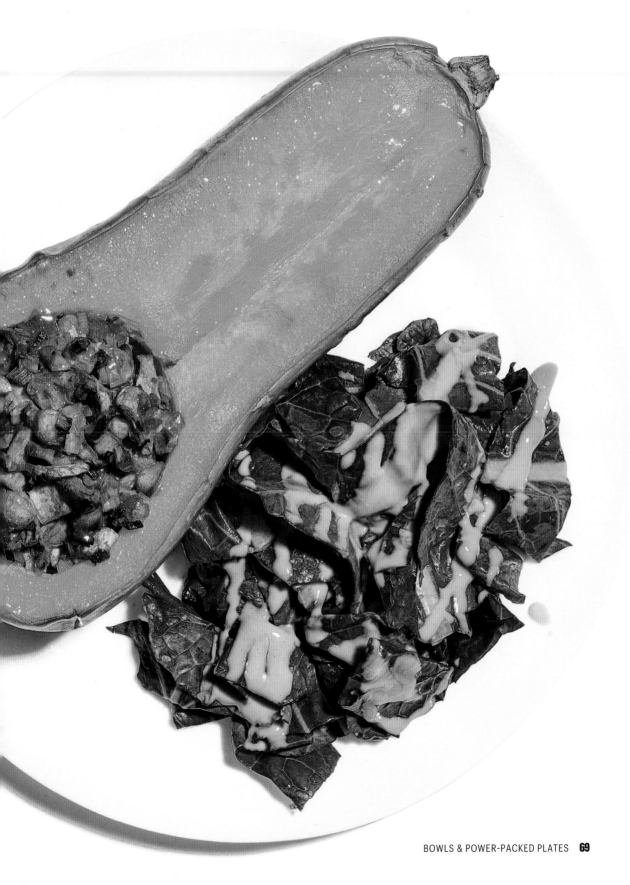

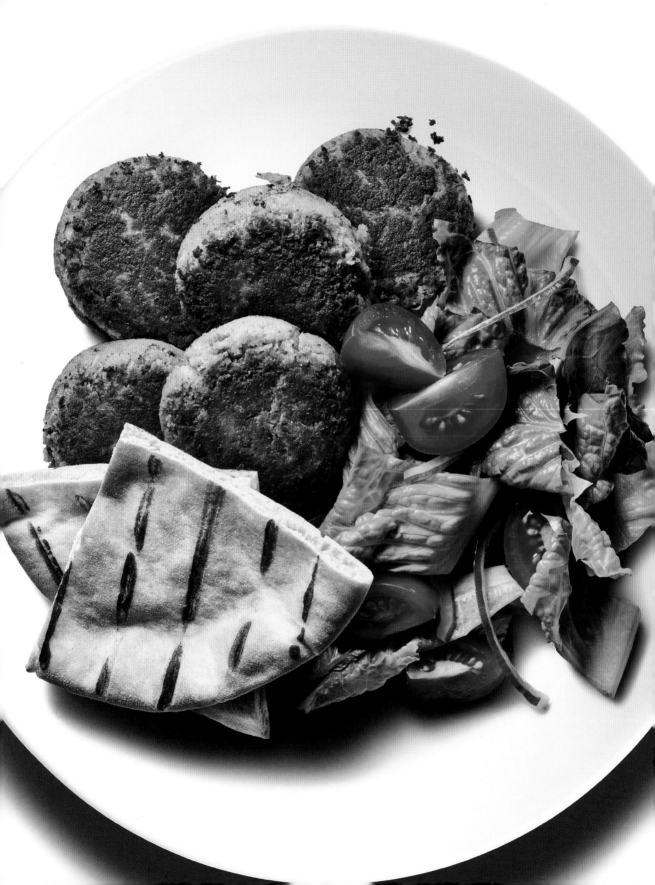

Deluxe Falafel Plate

SERVES 1

WHAT YOU'LL NEED:

1 (15 OZ) CAN CHICKPEAS, DRAINED

½ MEDIUM RED ONION, CHOPPED, PLUS MORE THINLY SLICED FOR SERVING

1 LARGE GARLIC CLOVE

¼ CUP FRESH PARSLEY LEAVES

1 TSP GROUND CUMIN

1 TBSP FRESH LEMON JUICE

¼ CUP BREAD CRUMBS

1 TSP BAKING POWDER

4 TBSP CANOLA OIL, PLUS MORE AS NEEDED

1 PITA, GRILLED OR WARMED

CHERRY TOMATOES, QUARTERED

CHOPPED LETTUCE

1. In a food processor, add the chickpeas, onion, garlic, parsley, cumin, lemon juice, ½ teaspoon each salt and pepper, bread crumbs, and baking powder. Pulse until mixture is well combined and looks like coarse crumbs.

2. Form falafel mixture into balls, using about 2 tablespoons for each ball. Gently flatten balls to about ½-inch thickness.

3. In a large cast-iron skillet heat 4 tablespoons oil over medium. Add 4 or 5 disks to the skillet and cook until browned and crisp, about 3 minutes per side. Transfer to a paper-towel-lined plate while cooking remaining falafel. Serve with pita, tomatoes, lettuce, and onion slices.

PER SERVING: *597 calories, 22 g protein, 51 g carbohydrates (9 g fiber), 36 g fat*

⫸ PROTEIN BOOST

Add protein with this easy sauce. Stir together ½ cup Greek yogurt, 1 tablespoon finely chopped fresh dill, and a squeeze of fresh lemon juice. Spoon over falafel.

GET A JUMP

You can make the falafel mixture up to three days ahead—and it will help when it comes to forming the balls. Just be sure to refrigerate in an airtight container.

Rosemary-Roasted Vegetables with Manchego Cheese and Serrano Ham

SERVES 1

WHAT YOU'LL NEED:

- ½ LB ASPARAGUS, TRIMMED AND CUT INTO 2-INCH PIECES
- ½ LB SMALL BRUSSELS SPROUTS, HALVED
- 2 TSP CHOPPED FRESH ROSEMARY
- 2 TSP OLIVE OIL
- 1 OZ SERRANO HAM, TORN INTO PIECES
- 1 TBSP SHERRY VINEGAR
- 2 TBSP SHAVED MANCHEGO CHEESE

1. Preheat your oven to 425°F. On a baking sheet, combine asparagus, Brussels sprouts, rosemary, oil, and a pinch of pepper.

2. Roast the vegetables, stirring once, until tender and just charred, about 20 minutes. Stir in ham and vinegar; roast for 2 minutes more.

3. Serve with cheese scattered on top.

PER SERVING: *322 calories, 21 g protein, 3 g carbohydrates (10 g fiber), 19 g fa*

⫘→ PROTEIN BOOST

Scatter ¼ cup sliced almonds, chopped walnuts, or pine nuts on the vegetables when you add the ham.

GREEN GIANT

Your eyes are not fooling you. The portion on this sheet pan may look massive, but it serves one. The idea is to bulk up on the vegetables (a pound total!) and treat the ham and cheese like sides.

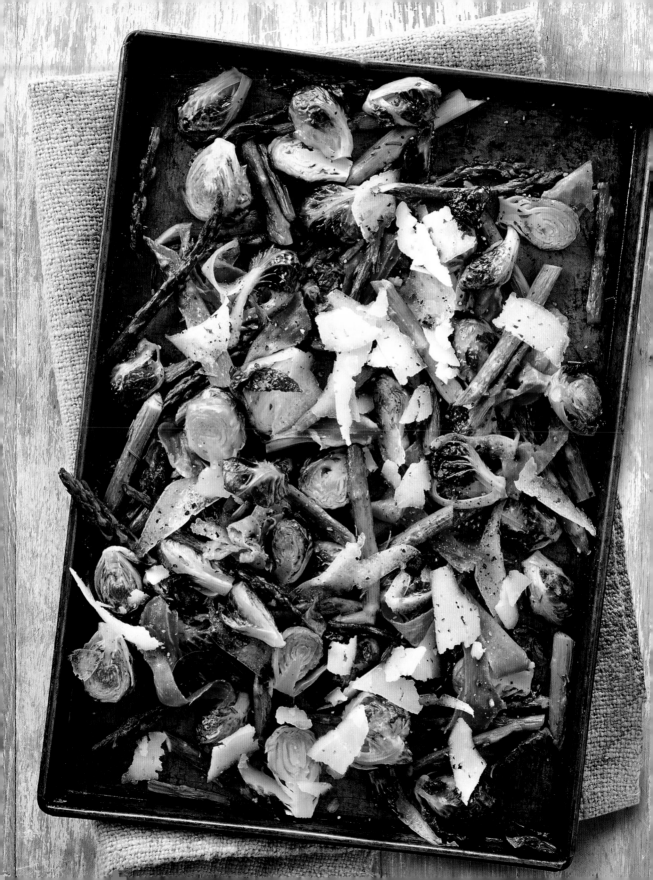

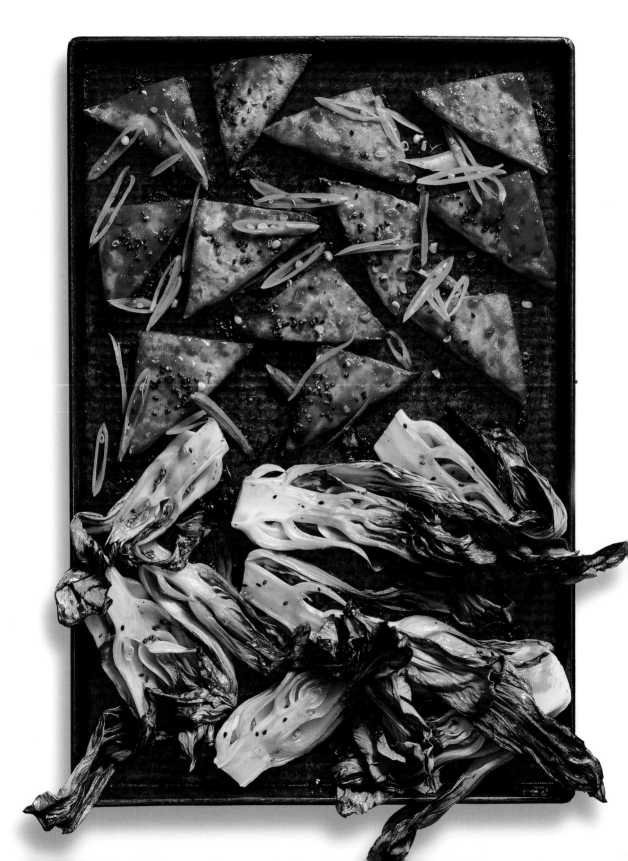

Asian Tofu with Baby Bok Choy

SERVES 2

WHAT YOU'LL NEED:

14 OZ EXTRA-FIRM TOFU, PRESSED BETWEEN PAPER TOWELS WITH A WEIGHT ON TOP FOR 30 MINUTES

4 TBSP SESAME GARLIC SAUCE (SUCH AS SIMPLY ENJOY), DIVIDED

8 HEADS BABY BOK CHOY, TRIMMED AND HALVED

2 TSP TOASTED SESAME OIL

1 TO 2 TSP SAMBAL OELEK HOT SAUCE OR SRIRACHA

4 SUGAR SNAP PEAS, THINLY SLICED

½ TSP BLACK SESAME SEEDS

1. Preheat your oven to 400°F. Slice tofu into ½-inch-thick triangles and arrange on half of a large lightly greased rimmed baking sheet. Drizzle with 1 tablespoon sesame garlic sauce and bake until top is golden, 10 to 12 minutes.

2. Remove from the oven, flip tofu, and drizzle with 1 tablespoon more sesame garlic sauce. Arrange bok choy on the other half of the sheet, and gently toss with sesame oil.

3. Return to the oven and bake until tofu is golden and bok choy is tender, about 10 minutes more.

4. Drizzle remaining 2 tablespoons sesame garlic sauce and the sambal oelek over tofu, and sprinkle with snap peas and sesame seeds.

PER SERVING: *316 calories, 26 g protein, 18 g carbohydrates (4 g fiber), 16 g fat*

A PAN FOR ALL SEASONS

Baking and roasting is only the beginning for your rimmed baking sheet. It also makes a perfectly acceptable pizza stone. Just invert and preheat in the oven—then slide your dough on top. Give it a try with Sunny Side Up Pizza on page 105, Marrakesh Express Pizza on page 106, or Spud Love Pizza on page 109.

Cauliflower Fried Rice

SERVES 4

WHAT YOU'LL NEED

- ½ LARGE HEAD CAULIFLOWER, CUT INTO FLORETS
- 2 TBSP VEGETABLE OIL, DIVIDED
- 1 ORANGE BELL PEPPER, SEEDED AND DICED
- 1 SCALLION, THINLY SLICED, WHITE AND GREEN PARTS SEPARATED
- 1 (2-INCH) PIECE FRESH GINGER, CUT INTO THIN MATCHSTICKS
- 2 TBSP LOW-SODIUM SOY SAUCE
- 2 TSP CHILI GARLIC PASTE
- 2 TSP HONEY
- 4 LARGE EGGS, LIGHTLY BEATEN
- 1 CUP FROZEN PEAS, THAWED
- 1 CUP FROZEN SHELLED EDAMAME, THAWED
- LIME WEDGES, FOR SERVING

1. Working in batches, pulse cauliflower in a food processor until the cauliflower resembles rice, about 15 seconds..

2. In a large cast-iron skillet over medium-high, heat 1 tablespoon oil. Add the pepper, the white parts of the scallion, and the ginger; cook, stirring, 2 minutes. Add the cauliflower, toss to combine, and cook, covered, stirring once, for 5 minutes.

3. Meanwhile, in a small bowl, whisk together the soy sauce, chili garlic paste, and honey. Push the cauliflower mixture to one side, add the remaining 1 tablespoon oil, then the eggs. Cook, stirring, until scrambled, about 2 minutes.

4. Remove the skillet from heat and fold in the sauce, peas, and edamame. Top servings with green parts of the scallion and serve with lime wedges.

PER SERVING: *251 calories, 15 g protein, 20 g carbohydrates (6 g fiber), 14 g fat*

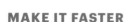 **PROTEIN BOOST**

Add 8 ounces thinly sliced leftover cooked beef, chicken, or pork when you fold in the peas.

MAKE IT FASTER

Swap the head of cauliflower for four cups cauliflower crumbles or rice.

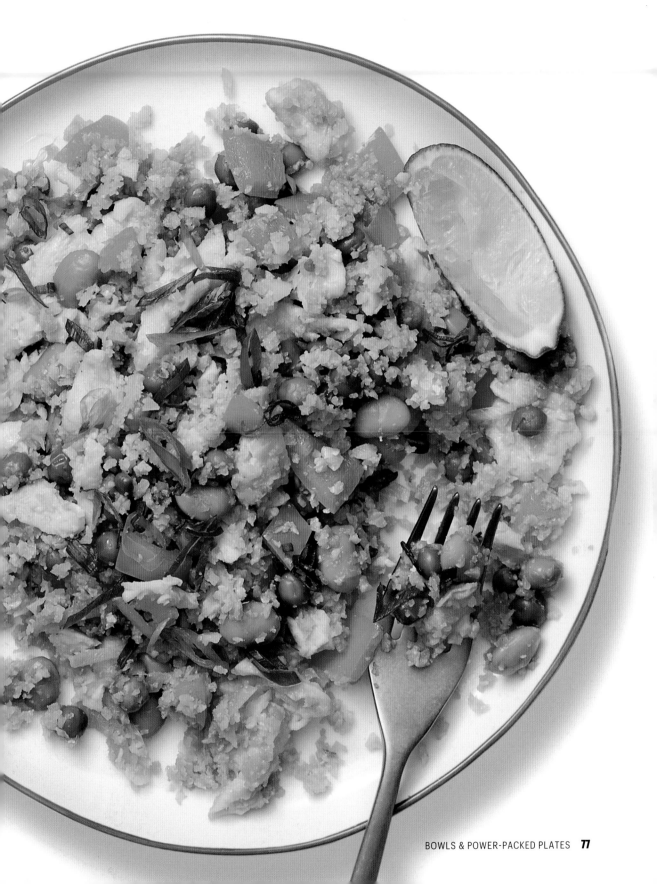

Power "Pasta" ❯

SERVES 1

WHAT YOU'LL NEED:

1 LARGE ZUCCHINI

1 CUP CHERRY TOMATOES

1 TBSP OLIVE OIL

1 CUP CHICKPEAS, DRAINED AND RINSED

1 SMALL COOKED BONELESS, SKINLESS CHICKEN THIGH, SLICED

¼ CUP TORN FRESH BASIL LEAVES

1. Use a vegetable spiral slicer or julienne peeler to cut the zucchini lengthwise into long strands.

2. In a large skillet, cook the zucchini and tomatoes in the olive oil over medium, turning carefully with tongs, until zucchini is just tender and tomato skins just begin to wrinkle and soften, 2 to 3 minutes. Add chickpeas and cook until heated through, 1 to 2 minutes.

3. Top zucchini, tomatoes, and chickpeas with chicken and basil.

PER SERVING: *350 calories, 33 g protein, 16 g carbohydrates (5 g fiber), 18 g fat*

Tofu Stir-Fry

SERVES 1

WHAT YOU'LL NEED:

1 TBSP CANOLA OIL

½ (14 OZ) BLOCK EXTRA-FIRM TOFU

½ CUP SHELLED EDAMAME

½ BUNCH ASPARAGUS, CHOPPED

1 CUP BROCCOLI FLORETS, CHOPPED

½ RED BELL PEPPER, SEEDED AND CHOPPED

½ CUP WATER CHESTNUTS, CHOPPED

½ CUP SUGAR SNAP PEAS, CHOPPED

RICE WINE VINEGAR

SOY SAUCE

In a large skillet over medium, heat the canola oil. Add the tofu, edamame, asparagus, broccoli, bell pepper, water chestnuts, and sugar snap peas, and cook, stirring frequently, until crisp-tender, 7 to 9 minutes. Season with a splash of rice wine vinegar and soy sauce.

PER SERVING: *530 calories, 35 g protein, 37 g carbohydrates (14 g fiber), 28 g fat*

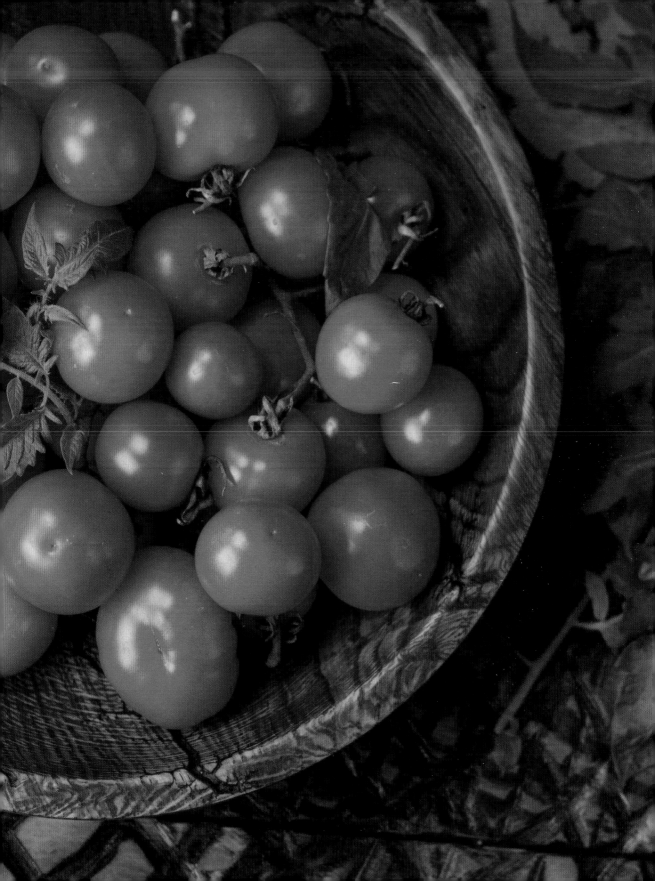

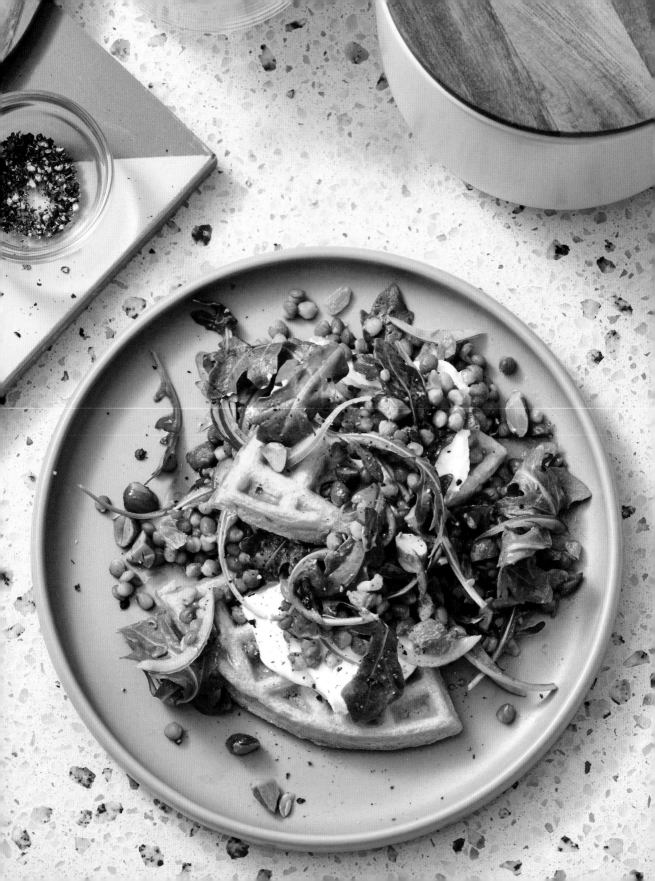

Savory Lentil Waffles

SERVES 4

WHAT YOU'LL NEED:

- 1 (14.5 OZ) CAN LENTILS, RINSED
- ¼ SMALL RED ONION, THINLY SLICED
- ¼ CUP GOLDEN RAISINS, CHOPPED
- 3 TBSP OLIVE OIL
- 3 TBSP SHERRY VINEGAR
- 1 CUP HIGH-PROTEIN PANCAKE AND WAFFLE MIX (SUCH AS KODIAK CAKES)
- 1 TSP CURRY POWDER
- ¼ TSP GROUND CORIANDER
- 4 CUPS BABY ARUGULA
- ¼ CUP TOASTED ALMONDS, CHOPPED
- GREEK YOGURT, FOR SERVING (OPTIONAL)

1. In a medium bowl, combine lentils, onion, raisins, oil, and vinegar.

2. In a large bowl, whisk together waffle mix, curry powder, coriander, and pinch each salt and pepper. Prepare two waffles in a waffle maker per manufacturer's directions.

3. When waffles are cooked, toss arugula and almonds with lentil mixture. Split waffles and spread with yogurt, if desired. Top with lentil salad.

PER SERVING: *362 calories, 16 g protein, 42 g carbohydrates (11 g fiber), 16 g fat*

⟶ PROTEIN BOOST

Eat these waffles ranchero-style with over-easy eggs and salsa.

PUMP UP SOME WAFFLE IRON

Who says waffles are just for breakfast? After you've tried these lentil-salad-topped beauties, try crispy waffles smothered in chili. Pairing them leftover with the Smoky Black Bean Chili on page 153 would give you the benefit of two legumes. Make waffle nachos or tacos with your favorite toppings.

Chana Saag with Greek Yogurt

SERVES 2

WHAT YOU'LL NEED:

- 1 TBSP CANOLA OIL
- ½ CUP DICED ONION
- 1 GARLIC CLOVE, MINCED
- 1 TSP CURRY POWDER
- 1 TSP GARAM MASALA
- 1 (14.5 OZ) CAN PETITE DICED TOMATOES, UNDRAINED
- 1 (15 OZ) CAN CHICKPEAS, DRAINED AND RINSED
- 5 OZ BABY SPINACH
- 2 CUPS PLAIN YOGURT

1. In a large skillet over medium-low, heat the oil. Add onion and garlic and cook until translucent, 5 to 6 minutes. Add curry powder and garam masala and cook until fragrant, about 1 minute.

2. Increase heat to medium and add tomatoes with juices, chickpeas, ¼ teaspoon each kosher salt and pepper; bring to a boil. Add spinach, stirring until wilted, 2 to 3 minutes.

3. Divide yogurt between two bowls and top with the chickpea mixture.

PER SERVING: *440 calories, 30 g protein, 50 g carbohydrates (14 g fiber), 14 g fat*

EAT YOUR GREENS

Saag refers to any greens-based Indian dish. This chana saag (chana is a type of chickpea) is a classic Indian curry made with chickpeas, loads of spinach, onion, tomato, ginger, garlic, curry powder, and garam masala. Curry powder, and some versions of garam masala, feature turmeric. Curcumin is the pigment that's responsible for the vivid yellow color of turmeric, and has been shown in studies to reduce inflammation and keep blood sugar levels steady.

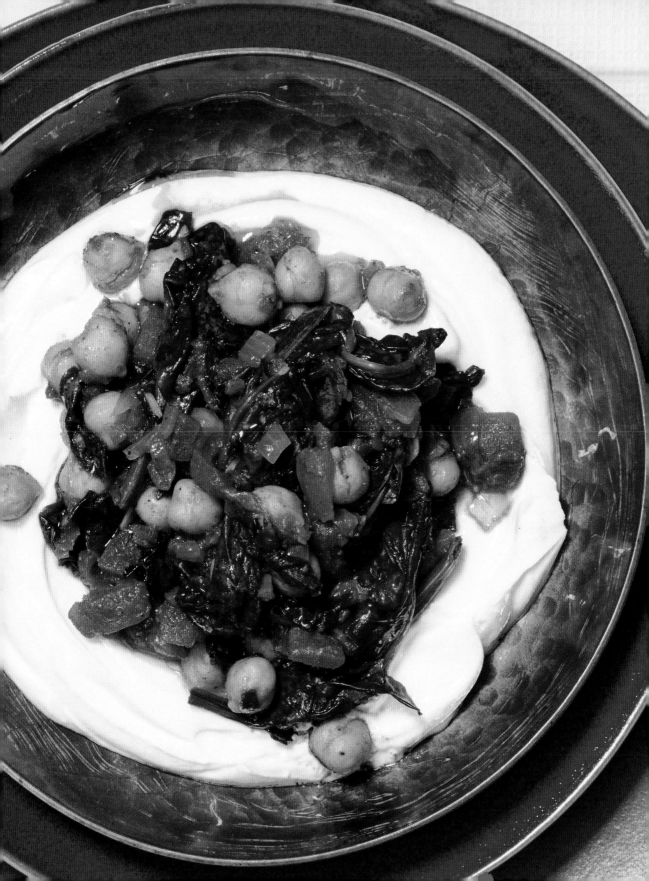

Red Peppers Stuffed with Tuscan Beans and Greens

SERVES 2

WHAT YOU'LL NEED:

- 4 OZ PANCETTA, DICED
- ½ SMALL ONION, DICED
- 1 GARLIC CLOVE, MINCED
- 1 (15 OZ) CAN WHITE BEANS, DRAINED
- 1 (14.5 OZ) CAN DICED TOMATOES, UNDRAINED
- ¼ CUP LOW-SODIUM CHICKEN BROTH
- ½ BUNCH KALE, STEMMED AND CHOPPED
- ½ CUP SMALL CROUTONS
- ¼ CUP GRATED PARMESAN
- 2 RED BELL PEPPERS, HALVED AND SEEDED

1. In a large skillet over medium, cook pancetta until it releases its oil. Add onion and garlic and cook until softened, about 3 minutes. Add beans, tomatoes, and chicken broth, and bring to a simmer.

2. Add kale; cover and cook until the kale is wilted, about 2 minutes. Stir in croutons and Parmesan. Spoon into pepper halves.

PER SERVING: 569 calories, 33 g protein, 68 g carbohydrates (24 g fiber), 19 g fat

TAKE A DIP

Blanching vegetables, the technique of giving them a quick dip in boiling water and then plunging them into a bowl of ice water to stop the cooking process, softens them slightly and brightens their color. If you blanch the bell pepper halves it will make them a bit more tender and they will retain a satisfying crunch.

Zucchini Stuffed with Quinoa Salad

SERVES 3

WHAT YOU'LL NEED:

3 ZUCCHINI, HALVED LENGTHWISE

¼ CUP OLIVE OIL

2 TBSP BALSAMIC VINEGAR

1 CUP COOKED QUINOA

½ CUP CANNED CHICKPEAS

1 SMALL RED ONION, DICED

1 RED BELL PEPPER, SEEDED AND DICED

¼ CUP CHOPPED PECANS

¼ CUP DRIED CRANBERRIES

2 TBSP CHOPPED FRESH PARSLEY

1. Use a spoon to scoop seeds out of zucchini halves, leaving a ½-inch shell. Discard seeds.

2. In a bowl, whisk oil, vinegar, 1 teaspoon salt, and ⅛ teaspoon pepper. Add quinoa, chickpeas, onion, bell pepper, pecans, dried cranberries, and parsley. Spoon filling into zucchini.

PER SERVING: *597 calories, 9 g protein, 44 g carbohydrates (8 g fiber), 45 g fat*

⊪⟶ **PROTEIN BOOST**

Serve with chicken and apple sausage— or go meatless with plant-based brats.

THE SUPERHERO GRAIN

Quinoa (KEEN-wah) has about twice as much protein as brown rice, and it's a complete protein and muscle-building powerhouse. With protein and fiber—plus healthy fats and a small dose of carbohydrates—the nutty seed also has a low impact on your blood sugar. It cooks just like rice; ready in about 15 minutes.

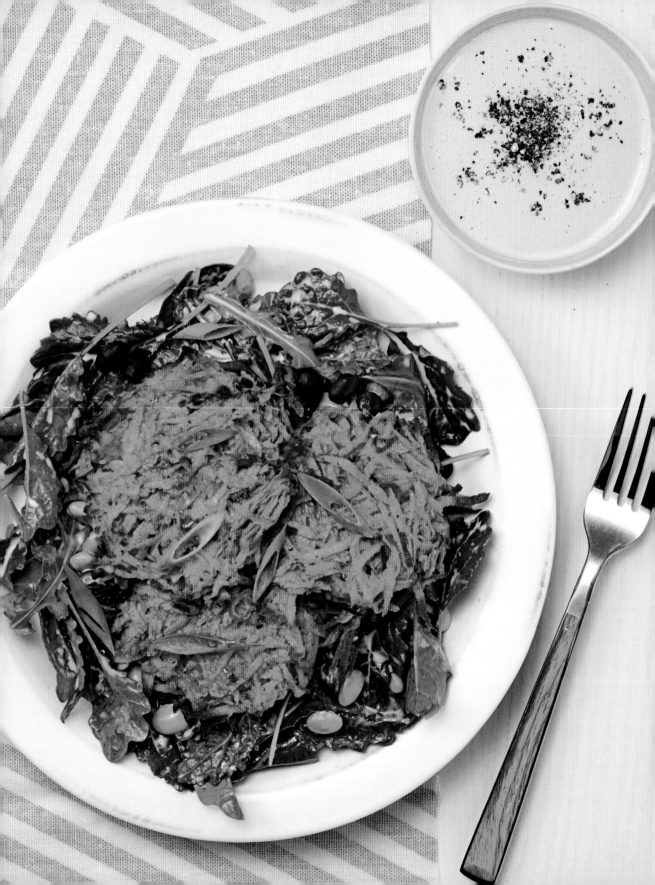

Sweet Potato Cakes with Kale and Bean Salad

SERVES 4

WHAT YOU'LL NEED:

COOKING SPRAY

3 SWEET POTATOES, PEELED AND SHREDDED

2 SCALLIONS, THINLY SLICED, PLUS MORE FOR SERVING

¼ CUP LIGHT MAYONNAISE

2 TBSP LIME JUICE

1 TBSP SOY SAUCE

5 OZ. BABY KALE

2 (14 OZ) CANS NO-SALT-ADDED BLACK BEANS, RINSED AND DRAINED

2 CUPS FROZEN SHELLED EDAMAME

1. Preheat your oven to 450°F. Coat a baking sheet with cooking spray.

2. In a large bowl, toss sweet potatoes, scallions, and ¼ teaspoon each salt and pepper. With a ¼-cup measuring cup, scoop sweet potatoes onto the baking sheet to form 12 mounds, 2 inches apart. Flatten slightly. Spray tops with cooking spray. Bake 25 minutes or until browned at edges.

3. In another large bowl, whisk mayonnaise, lime juice, and soy sauce. Toss the baby kale, black beans, and edamame with the dressing until coated. Serve the cakes over salad, and top with a few scallions.

PER SERVING: *375 calories, 21 g protein, 56 g carbohydrates (16 g fiber), 9 g fat*

⫿⟶ **PROTEIN BOOST**

Add more protein with a sweet treat: Chocolately Clusters on page 206.

HEALTHY GREENS IN A HEARTBEAT

Take a tub of hearty leafy greens—baby kale, spinach, chard or a mix—dump it in a wok coated with a glug or two of olive oil, turn the heat to high and then stir for five minutes. What remains is sauteed greens that are tender and delicious. Dress them with a little salt and pepper, and that's it. The nutritional benefit of this method is huge. *Men's Health* recommends two to four servings of leafy greens a day. When you "wok" an entire tub of greens, you can eat 3½ servings in one sitting, no sweat.

Build a Better Bowl

More people are saying that quality tops convenience when it comes to fast food. And while you could visit healthy-eating havens, you could also just steal their best ideas. Enter the bowl.

Healthy bowls—those fresh, customized meals that combine all sorts of greens, grains, vegetables, legumes, squash, and berries—are a layered masterpiece in all things delicious. Need help getting started? Pick one or two options for each layer.

The smaller you cut your ingredients, the faster they cook and the more they absorb other flavors. Dice proteins and produce smaller than bite-size.

BOTTOM LAYER

Flimsy greens get soggy when dressed. For make-and-take bowls, opt for sturdier fare.

Shredded: kale, Brussels sprouts, broccoli, cabbage

Zoodled: zucchini, yellow squash, carrots, beets

Riced: cauliflower, broccoli

Cooked: quinoa, farro, sweet potato, lentils

MIDDLE LAYER

There's more to building muscle than grilled chicken. These options are packed with protein and flavor: **crispy chickpeas, pan-fried falafel, grilled tempeh, marinated tofu, edamame.**

TOP LAYER

Quick-pickled: radishes, shiitake mushrooms, jicama, red onions, cucumbers, mangoes

Grilled: avocados, pineapples, peaches, plums, bell peppers, scallions

Roasted: mushrooms, beets, sweet potatoes, red peppers, corn kernels, chickpeas

Straight-up: diced apples, berries, diced dates, dried cranberries, dried cherries, pita chips, chopped fresh mint, bean sprouts

THE SAUCE

Bottled supermarket salad dressings often hit one note—sweet. Instead, make your own. Get ahead for the week and batch-prep sauces. Just pour a few portions into ice-cube trays and freeze. Microwave a cube to defrost it quickly. For recipes, see right page.

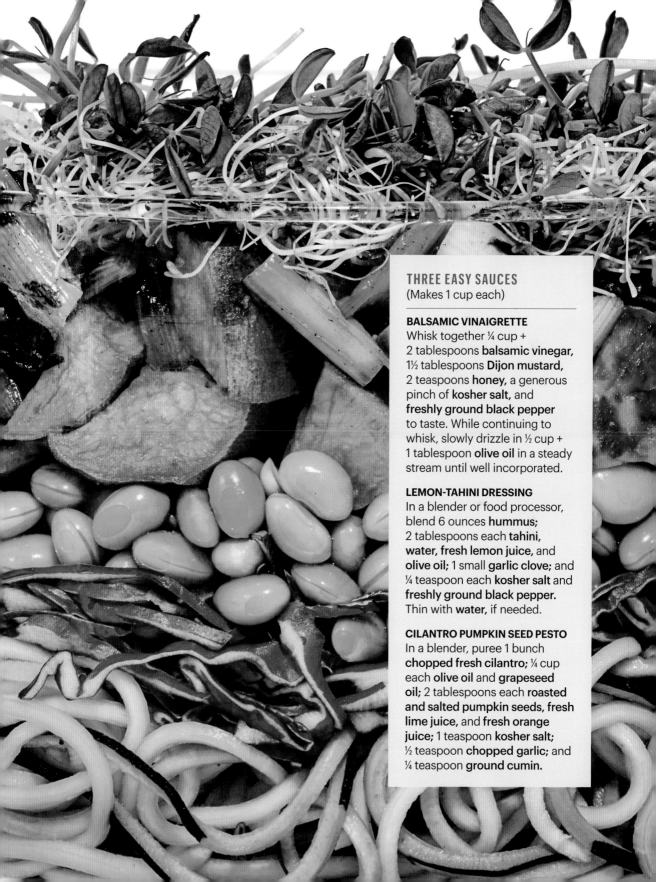

THREE EASY SAUCES
(Makes 1 cup each)

BALSAMIC VINAIGRETTE
Whisk together ¼ cup +
2 tablespoons **balsamic vinegar,**
1½ tablespoons **Dijon mustard,**
2 teaspoons **honey,** a generous
pinch of **kosher salt,** and
freshly ground black pepper
to taste. While continuing to
whisk, slowly drizzle in ½ cup +
1 tablespoon **olive oil** in a steady
stream until well incorporated.

LEMON-TAHINI DRESSING
In a blender or food processor,
blend 6 ounces **hummus;**
2 tablespoons each **tahini,**
water, fresh lemon juice, and
olive oil; 1 small **garlic clove;** and
¼ teaspoon each **kosher salt** and
freshly ground black pepper.
Thin with **water,** if needed.

CILANTRO PUMPKIN SEED PESTO
In a blender, puree 1 bunch
chopped fresh cilantro; ¼ cup
each **olive oil** and **grapeseed**
oil; 2 tablespoons each **roasted**
and salted pumpkin seeds, fresh
lime juice, and **fresh orange**
juice; 1 teaspoon **kosher salt;**
½ teaspoon **chopped garlic;** and
¼ teaspoon **ground cumin.**

Burgers, Sandwiches & Tacos

Going plant-based does not mean you have to give up on your favorite foods. It also doesn't mean that you have to replace your favorite foods with lesser versions either. (Because, honestly, who ever tasted a Portobello mushroom burger and said, "You know what? I'm done with beef.") Instead, think of these plant-forward spins on old standbys as new additions to your lineup.

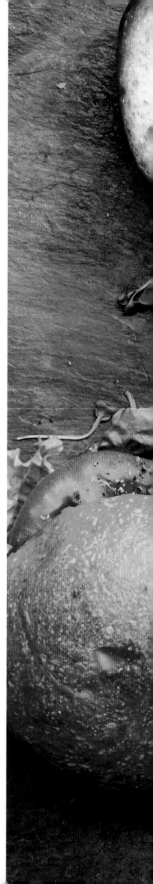

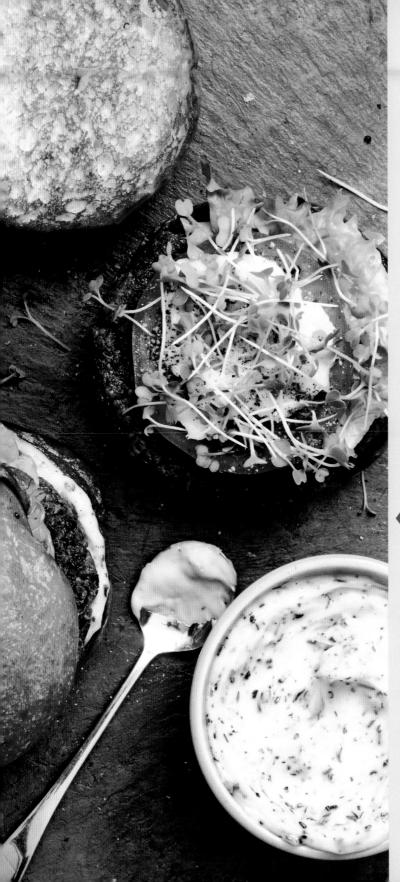

THE RECIPES

"B"LT

SERVES 2

WHAT YOU'LL NEED:

1 (8 OZ) PACKAGE TEMPEH, THINLY SLICED

3 TBSP SOY SAUCE

1 TBSP LIQUID SMOKE

1 TBSP CANOLA OIL

1 TBSP MAYONNAISE

2 TSP HOT SAUCE, SUCH AS SRIRACHA

4 SLICES SOURDOUGH, TOASTED

½ AVOCADO, PITTED AND PEELED

1 TOMATO, THINLY SLICED

2 ROMAINE LEAVES

1. In a zip-top bag, combine the tempeh, soy sauce, and liquid smoke. Refrigerate for at least 1 hour or up to 4 hours.

2. In a large skillet over medium-high, heat the oil. Add the tempeh and cook until browned, 1 to 2 minutes on each side. Transfer to a plate.

3. In a small bowl, mix the mayo and hot sauce. Slather one side of two slices of bread with spicy mayo. Mash the avocado half onto one side of the two other slices of bread. Layer each sandwich with tempeh, tomato, and lettuce.

PER SERVING: *758 calories, 36 g protein, 89 g carbohydrates (7 g fiber), 31 g fat*

YEAH, IT'S NOT BACON, BUT...

Marinated tempeh—a textured soy protein that's denser and meatier than tofu—stands in for bacon in this stacked sandwich. Tempeh is more protein-packed and vitamin-dense than tofu—and, it's more firm, flavorful, and meatlike. It has a whopping 20 grams of protein and five grams of fiber in just four ounces. Made from cooked, cracked soybeans, tempeh usually includes a grain, such as millet, brown rice, or barley, and sometimes all three. Tempeh is sold in the refrigerated section of the supermarket.

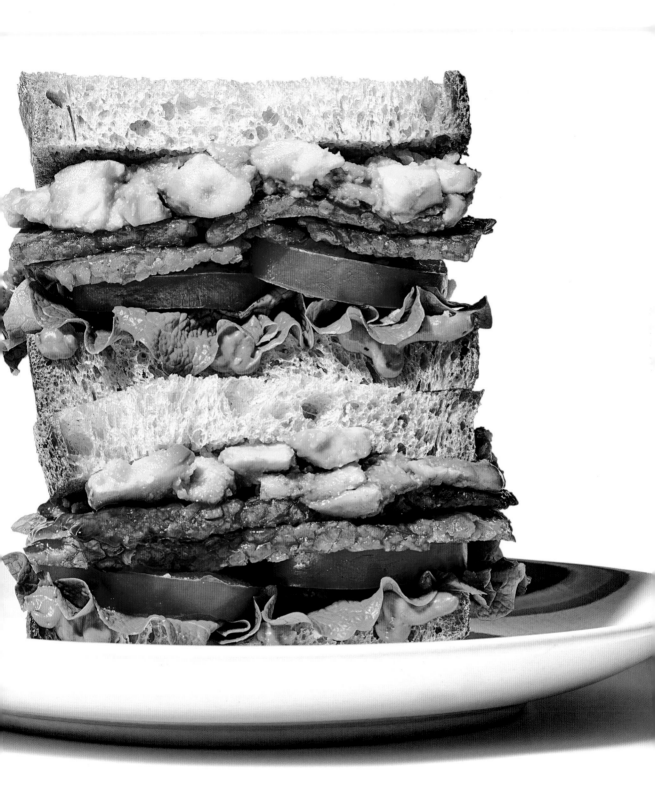

That's a Wrap

Here's how this works: Pick a leafy wrap for your base, fill it with a protein, and add a topping mix. Then wrap and eat. These combos make four wraps, or two servings total. You can prepare the ingredients ahead of time, then assemble the wraps when you're ready to eat or pack your lunch.

LEAFY OPTIONS

Bibb Lettuce: This tender lettuce is very pliable and has a mild flavor. It's best for light-weight fillings.

Radicchio Leaves: The sturdy leaves have a bitter edge. They're good combined with strong flavored foods.

Green Cabbage: Fresh and lightly peppery, these super crunchy leaves serve best as a cup for the filling.

Napa Cabbage: The elongated leaves are ruffly and tender.

Greens: The sturdy leaves can hold their own against hearty fillings. They do need to be blanched before using.

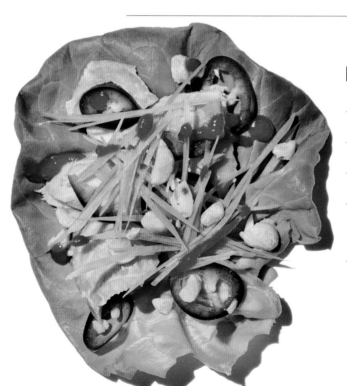

1 THAI CRUNCH WRAPS

WHAT YOU'LL NEED:

- 8 BIBB LETTUCE LEAVES
- 4 OZ COOKED SALMON, FLAKED
- ½ CUP CHOPPED SALTED PEANUTS
- 1 CUP SHREDDED CARROTS
- ¼ CUP THINLY SLICED JALAPEÑO PEPPERS
- SRIRACHA SAUCE

Place the Bibb lettuce leaves on a work surface, and top with the flaked salmon, chopped peanuts, shredded carrots, jalapeño slices, and sriracha sauce to taste. Serves 2.

PER SERVING:
327 calories, 25 g protein, 13 g carbohydrates (5 g fiber), 22 g fat

2 TEX-MEX WRAPS

WHAT YOU'LL NEED:

2½ CUPS COOKED QUINOA

1¾ CUPS BLACK BEANS, RINSED AND DRAINED

1 AVOCADO, PITTED, PEELED, AND DICED

1 MEDIUM TOMATO, DICED

2 TBSP CHOPPED FRESH CILANTRO

JUICE FROM 1 LIME

CAYENNE PEPPER, TO TASTE

8 RADICCHIO LEAVES

In a bowl, mix quinoa, black beans, avocado, tomato, cilantro, lime juice, ¼ teaspoon salt, and cayenne pepper. Place the radicchio leaves on a work surface, and top with the black bean mixture. Serves 2.

PER SERVING:
644 calories, 26 g protein, 100 g carbohydrates (27 g fiber), 20 g fat

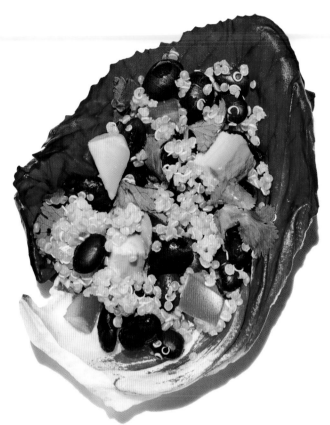

3 HIPPIE-STYLE CHICKEN WRAPS

WHAT YOU'LL NEED:

8 COLLARD GREENS LEAVES, STEMS TRIMMED

1¼ CUPS HUMMUS

3 TBSP SRIRACHA SAUCE

4 OZ CUBED ROTISSERIE CHICKEN

½ CUP THINLY SLICED RED ONION

1½ CUPS ALFALFA SPROUTS

Bring a large pot of water to a boil and add the leaves. Boil for 5 minutes, then dunk into a large bowl of ice water until cool. Dry the leaves. In a bowl, stir together hummus and sriracha. Spoon onto leaves, then add the chicken, red onion, and alfalfa sprouts. Serves 2.

PER SERVING:
388 calories, 25 g protein, 33 g carbohydrates (13 g fiber), 23 g fat

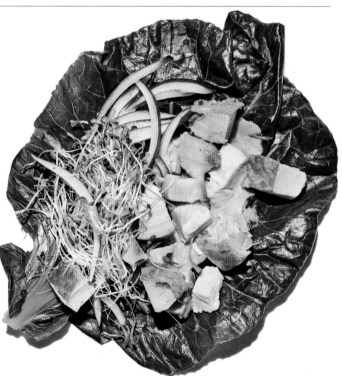

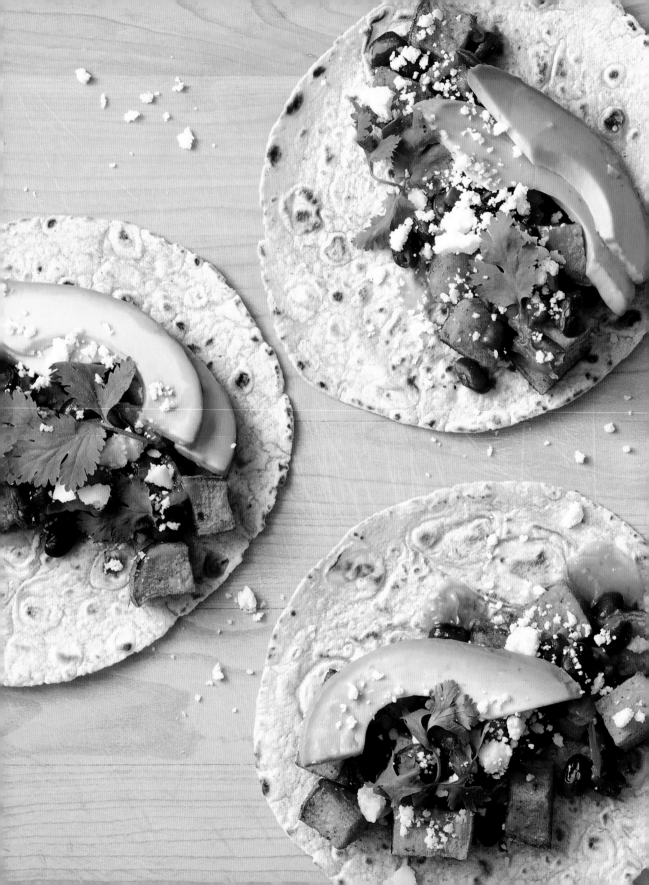

Sweet Potato and Black Bean Tacos

SERVES 4

WHAT YOU'LL NEED:

1¼ LB SWEET POTATOES, SCRUBBED AND CUT INTO ½-INCH CHUNKS

1 TBSP OLIVE OIL

1 TSP CHILI POWDER

1 (15 OZ) CAN NO-SALT-ADDED BLACK BEANS, DRAINED AND RINSED

½ CUP SALSA VERDE

8 FLOUR OR CORN TORTILLAS, WARMED

1 AVOCADO, PITTED, PEELED, AND THINLY SLICED

¼ CUP CRUMBLED FETA CHEESE

FRESH CILANTRO, FOR TOPPING

1. Preheat your oven to 450°F. Toss the sweet potatoes with olive oil, chili powder, and ½ teaspoon salt. Arrange on a large rimmed baking sheet; roast for 30 minutes.

2. In a saucepan, combine the black beans with the salsa verde; heat on medium until warm, stirring frequently.

3. Spoon the sweet potatoes and beans onto the tortillas, and top with avocado slices, cheese, and cilantro.

PER SERVING: *465 calories, 13 g protein, 70 g carbohydrates (16 g fiber), 16 g fat*

⊪→ PROTEIN BOOST

Add ¼ cup diced cooked chicken, beef, or tempeh to each taco.

THE MIGHTY BLACK BEAN

A staple in Mexican cuisine, black beans are a good source of iron, phosphorus, calcium, magnesium, potassium, copper, zinc, and fiber. If you have the time to buy dried beans and soak them, the texture is worth it. But canned beans work in a pinch too. Just remember to rinse them well to remove excess starch.

Mushroom Quinoa Burgers with Rosemary Mayo

SERVES 4

WHAT YOU'LL NEED:

4 MEDIUM PORTOBELLO MUSHROOM CAPS (ABOUT 1 LB), GILLS REMOVED, CHOPPED

½ CUP WALNUTS

1 GARLIC CLOVE

2 TBSP CANOLA OIL, DIVIDED

¼ CUP CHOPPED RED ONION

3 SCALLIONS, CHOPPED

2 TSP RICE WINE VINEGAR

1 CUP COOKED QUINOA

½ CUP CORNSTARCH

½ CUP MAYONNAISE

1 TSP FINELY CHOPPED FRESH ROSEMARY

1 TSP LEMON JUICE

4 WHOLE-GRAIN BUNS, TOASTED

SPROUTS, LETTUCE, AND SLICED TOMATO, FOR SERVING

1. Preheat your oven to 375°F. In a 3-quart baking dish, toss the mushrooms with walnuts, garlic, 1 tablespoon oil, ¾ teaspoon salt, and ¼ teaspoon pepper, then spread in an even layer. Bake until the mushrooms are tender, 20 minutes. Set aside to cool.

2. In a food processor, pulse the mushroom mixture, onion, scallions, and vinegar until mostly smooth. Transfer the mixture to a large bowl and stir in quinoa and cornstarch. Cover the bowl with plastic wrap and refrigerate for 2 hours.

3. Preheat your oven to 375°F. Line a baking sheet with foil. Form the mushroom mixture into four patties (about ½-inch thick and 3-inch wide). In a 12-inch nonstick skillet over medium, heat the remaining 1 tablespoon oil. In 2 batches, cook the patties until well-browned, about 5 minutes, turning over once. Transfer the seared patties to the baking sheet. Bake until heated through, about 10 minutes.

4. For the rosemary mayo, in a small bowl, combine mayonnaise, rosemary, lemon juice, and a pinch of salt.

5. Serve the burgers on buns with rosemary mayo, topped with sprouts, lettuce, and tomato.

PER SERVING: *495 calories, 9 g protein, 49 g carbohydrates (7 g fiber), 31 g fat*

|||→ **PROTEIN BOOST**

Serve the burgers with the Vegetable Trio on Sweet Mash on page 170.

GET AHEAD OF THE CURVE

You know how it goes: You get home from the gym and you want to eat—now. This is when a little planning pays off. The mushroom mixture can be made a couple of days ahead, along with the rosemary mayo.

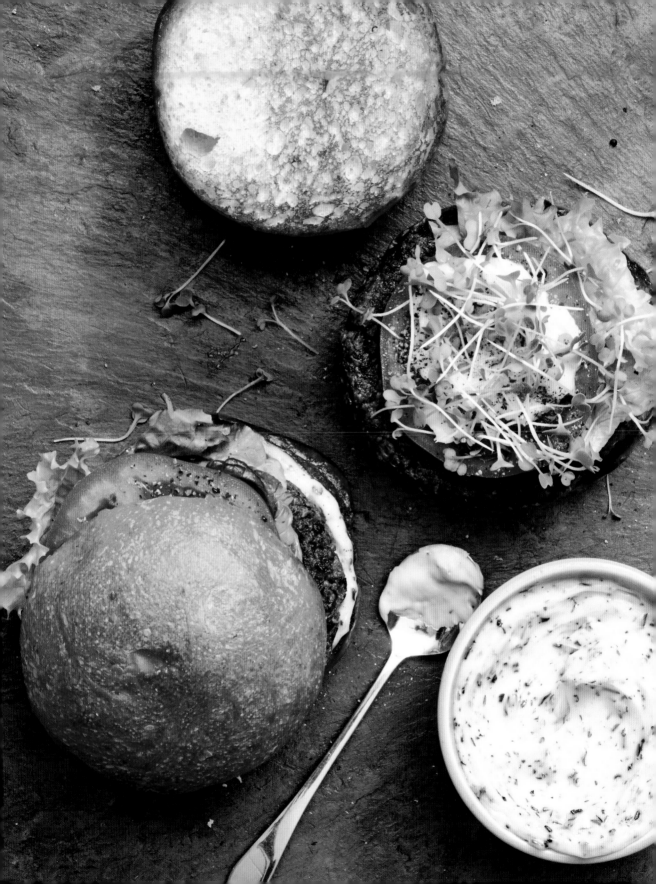

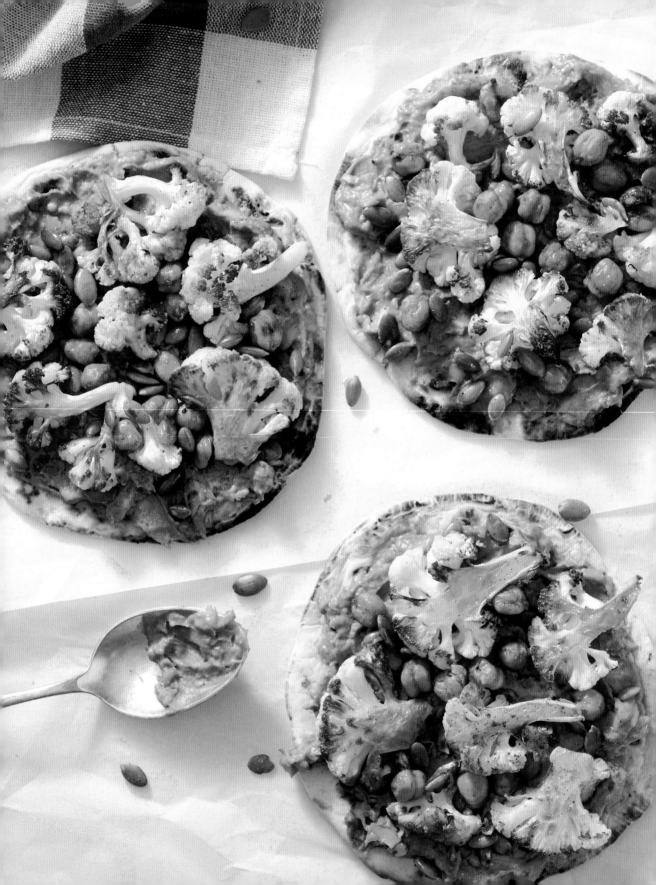

BBQ Chickpea and Cauliflower Flatbreads with Avocado Mash

SERVES 4

WHAT YOU'LL NEED:

- 12 OZ SMALL CAULIFLOWER FLORETS
- 1 TBSP OLIVE OIL
- 2 AVOCADOS, HALVED, PITTED, AND PEELED
- JUICE FROM 1 LEMON
- 4 FLATBREADS OR POCKETLESS PITAS, TOASTED
- ½ CUP CHICKPEA "NUTS" ON PAGE 205
- 2 TBSP SALTED ROASTED PEPITAS
- HOT SAUCE, FOR SERVING

1. Preheat your oven to 425°F. On a large rimmed baking sheet, toss together the cauliflower, olive oil, and ¼ teaspoon salt. Roast until tender and browned, about 25 minutes.

2. Mash avocados with lemon juice and a pinch salt; spread all over flatbreads. Top with roasted cauliflower, chickpeas, and pepitas. Serve with hot sauce.

PER SERVING: *499 calories, 11 g protein, 64 g carbohydrates (13 g fiber), 25 g fat*

||⟶ **PROTEIN BOOST**

Add a side of Shredded Brussels Sprouts with Pistachios and Prosciutto on page 181.

SMALL BUT MIGHTY

Antioxidant-rich pepitas—the seeds of specific types of pumpkins that don't require shelling—are loaded with magnesium, zinc, fiber, and protein. Eat 'em raw or roasted, tossed on salads, soups, and flatbreads.

Fish on Rye

SERVES 1

WHAT YOU'LL NEED:
2 OZ COOKED SALMON, FLAKED
1 TBSP MAYONNAISE
¼ CUP MINCED CELERY
JUICE OF 1 LIME
½ CUP NAVY BEANS
2 SLICES DARK RYE BREAD

Mash together the salmon, mayonnaise, celery, lime juice, and navy beans. Pile between bread slices.

PER SERVING: *451 calories, 25 g protein, 54 g carbohydrates (12 g fiber), 15 g fat*

Brat Rolls >

SERVES 1

WHAT YOU'LL NEED:
1 WHOLE-WHEAT STEAK ROLL, SPLIT AND GRILLED OR TOASTED
¾ CUP SAUERKRAUT, WARMED
1 GRILLED BEYOND BRAT
SPICY BROWN MUSTARD

Top the steak roll with sauerkraut then add the brat. Top with mustard.

PER SERVING: *654 calories, 30 g protein, 72 g carbohydrates (15 g fiber), 27 g fat*

SUDS, ON THE SIDE

You know what goes great with both of these sandwiches? Beer. And if you really think about it, hops and malts are plant-based. So beer is plant-based. *Mmmmm* delicious plant-based beer.

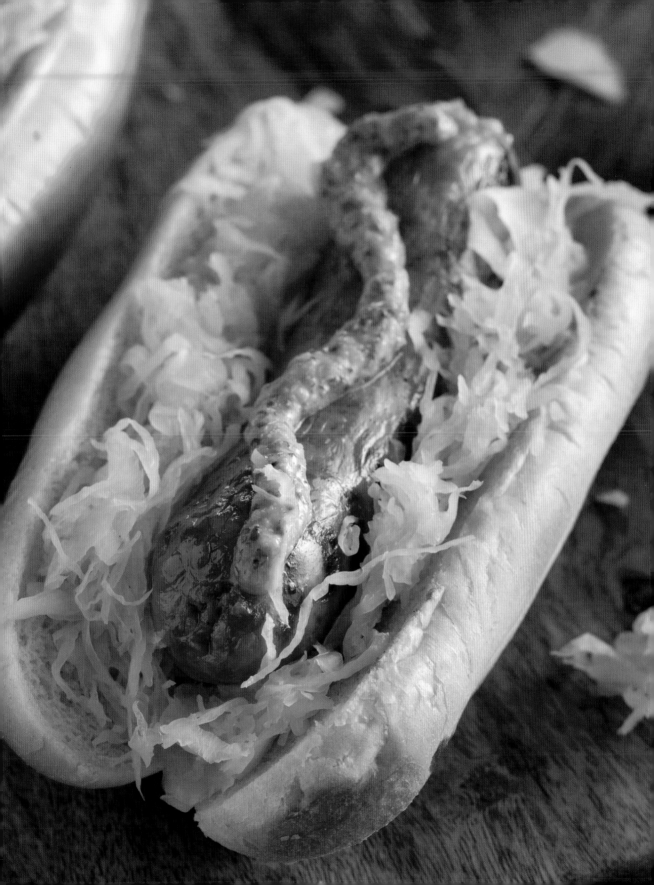

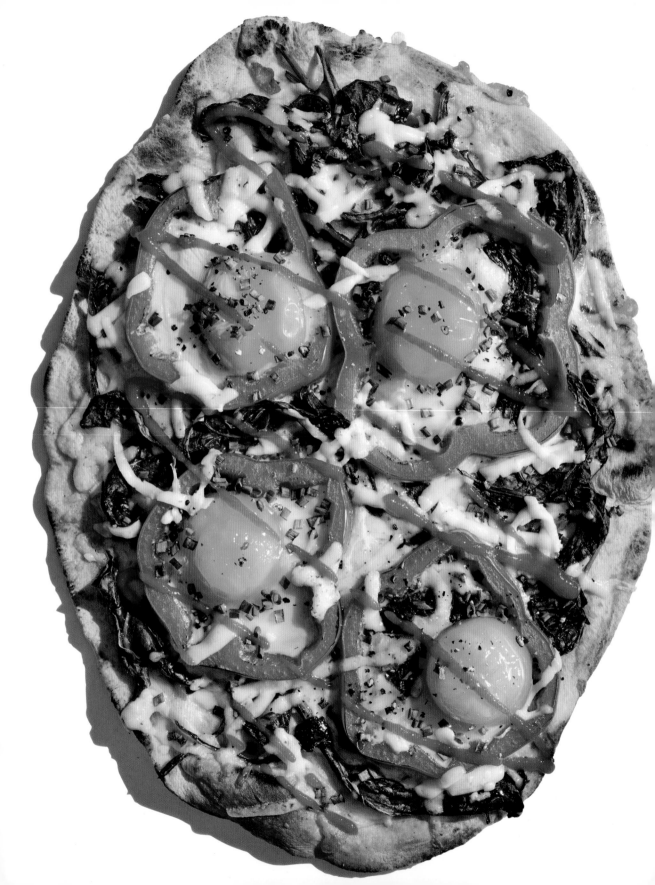

Sunny Side Up Pizza

SERVES 4

WHAT YOU'LL NEED:

- 1 1-LB BALL OF PIZZA CRUST DOUGH
- 1 TBSP OIL
- ½ CUP TOMATO SAUCE
- 2 CUPS FRESH BABY SPINACH
- 1 CUP SHREDDED HAVARTI CHEESE
- 4 RED BELL PEPPER RINGS
- 4 EGGS
- CHOPPED FRESH CHIVES
- HOT SAUCE

1. On a lightly floured surface, stretch and/or roll the dough until about ½-inch thick. (The shape doesn't matter as long as the dough fits on your grill.)

2. Preheat your grill to indirect medium heat. Lightly oil the grill grates. Set up a work area nearby with your toppings in reach.

3. Brush one side of the dough with oil. Place that side over indirect heat and grill until lightly charred, 1 to 2 minutes. Flip the dough onto the work area, cooked side up.

4. Spread the tomato sauce on the crust, then add the spinach, havarti, and peppers. Carefully crack eggs on top inside the pepper rings, and return the pizza to indirect heat. Close the grill lid and cook until the edges are crispy and egg whites are set, 5 to 7 minutes. Top with chives and hot sauce; allow to cool a few minutes, then slice.

PER SERVING: *481 calories, 20 g protein, 52 g carbohydrates (3 g fiber), 20 g fat*

||—▶ **PROTEIN BOOST**

Top pizza with 6 slices regular or plant-based crisp-cooked and crumbled bacon to meet your 25 grams of protein goal.

SCORE DOUGH

Most grocery stores carry one-pound balls of pizza dough—if you're lucky, they'll have a whole-wheat option as well. You can also ask your neighborhood pizzeria if they'll sell you their pizza dough. You can even get multiples and freeze them. Just put each ball of dough in its own resealable plastic freezer bag and freeze up to three months. Take it out of the freezer and put it in the refrigerator the morning of the day you want to use it. Then roll, top, and grill/bake as usual.

Marrakesh Express Pizza

SERVES 4

WHAT YOU'LL NEED:

- 1 1-LB BALL OF PIZZA CRUST DOUGH
- 1 TBSP OIL
- ½ CUP PURCHASED BABA GHANOUSH
- 8 OZ CRUMBLED COOKED SAUSAGE
- 1 CUP SLICED GRILLED YELLOW SUMMER SQUASH
- ½ CUP SLICED PIQUILLO PEPPER OR ROASTED RED BELL PEPPERS
- ¼ CUP SLICED BLACK OLIVES
- 1 CUP SHREDDED GRUYÈRE CHEESE
- FENNEL SEEDS, TOASTED

1. On a lightly floured surface, stretch and/or roll the dough until about ½-inch thick. (The shape doesn't matter as long as the dough fits on your grill.)

2. Preheat your grill to indirect medium heat. Lightly oil the grill grates. Set up a work area nearby with your toppings in reach.

3. Brush one side of the dough with oil. Place that side over indirect heat and grill until lightly charred, 1 to 2 minutes. Flip the dough onto the work area, cooked side up.

4. Spread the baba ghanoush on the crust, then add the sausage, summer squash, peppers, olives, and Gruyère, and return the pizza to indirect heat. Close the grill lid and cook until the edges are crispy, 5 to 7 minutes. Sprinkle with fennel feeds; allow to cool a few minutes, then slice.

PER SERVING: *677 calories, 28 g protein, 60 g carbohydrates (6 g fiber), 36 g fat*

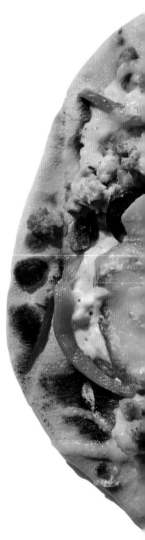

PREP THE FIXINGS

Grill vegetables like zucchini, summer squash, eggplant, bell peppers, onions, and mushrooms before assembling your pie. If added raw, most produce won't become tender while the pizza cooks. All raw meats must be cooked before topping the pizza.

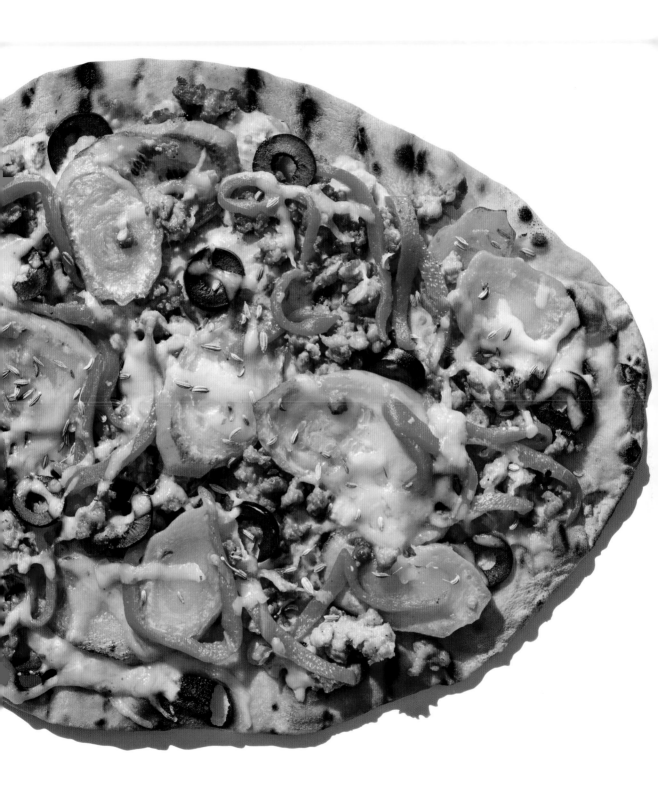

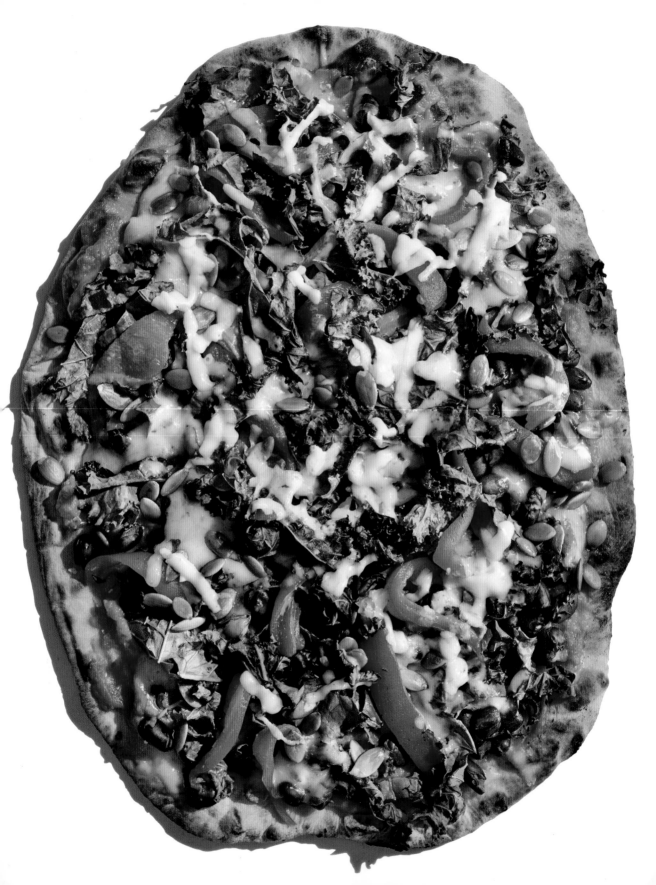

Spud Love Pizza

SERVES 4

WHAT YOU'LL NEED:

1 1-LB BALL OF PIZZA CRUST DOUGH

1 TBSP OIL

½ CUP SWEET POTATO PUREE

2 CUPS CHOPPED KALE

¾ CUP BLACK BEANS

½ CUP SLICED ROASTED RED PEPPERS

1 CUP SHREDDED FONTINA CHEESE

PEPITAS

1. On a lightly floured surface, stretch and/or roll the dough until about ½-inch thick. (The shape doesn't matter as long as the dough fits on your grill.)

2. Preheat your grill to indirect medium heat. Lightly oil the grill grates. Set up a work area nearby with your toppings in reach.

3. Brush one side of the dough with oil. Place that side over indirect heat and grill until lightly charred, 1 to 2 minutes. Flip the dough onto the work area, cooked side up.

4. Spread the sweet potato puree onto the crust. Top with the kale, black beans, peppers, and Fontina cheese, and return the pizza to indirect heat. Close the grill lid and cook until the edges are crispy, 5 to 7 minutes. Sprinkle with pepitas; allow to cool a few minutes, then slice.

PER SERVING: *497 calories, 19 g protein, 69 g carbohydrates (9 g fiber), 17 g fat*

⫸ PROTEIN BOOST

Scatter 1 cup leftover chicken or plant-based meat crumbles along with the other toppings.

PERSONAL PIZZA

DIY pizza is fresher and can reflect your mood. Not feeling this combination? Change it up with a different spread (refried beans, BBQ sauce, marinara sauce, or pesto), toppings (halved cherry tomatoes, mixed mushrooms, artichoke hearts), and cheese (Gouda, provolone, mozzarella, Jack).

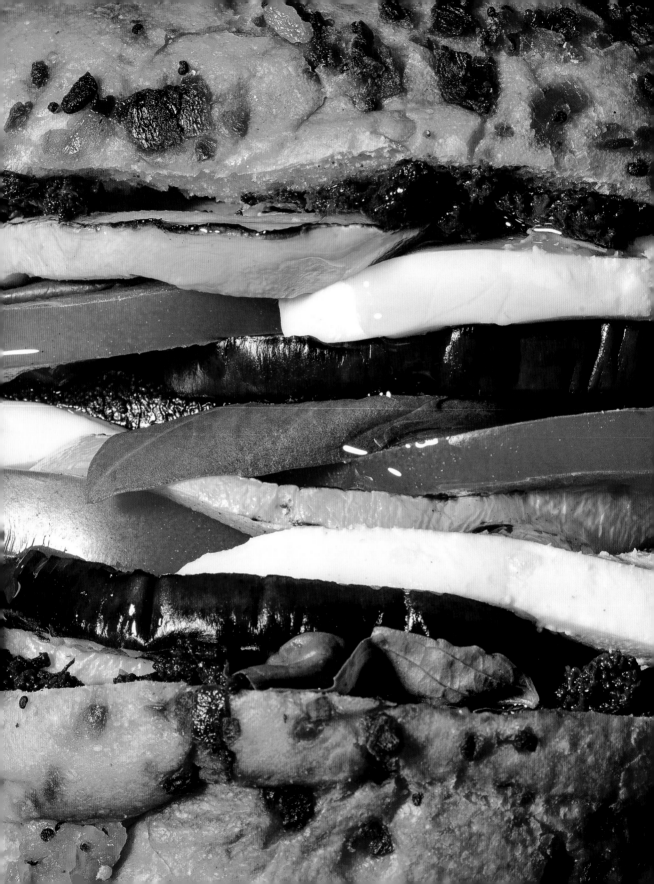

Ratatouille Royale

SERVES 1

WHAT YOU'LL NEED:

¼ CUP KALAMATA OLIVE TAPENADE

1 ONION ROLL, SPLIT AND GRILLED OR TOASTED

2 OZ FRESH MOZZARELLA, SLICED

2 SLICES GRILLED EGGPLANT

2 LONG SLICES GRILLED YELLOW SQUASH

2 LONG SLICES GRILLED ZUCCHINI

4 TOMATO SLICES

FRESH BASIL LEAVES

Spread half of the olive tapenade on the onion roll bottom, then layer half the mozzarella, eggplant, yellow squash, zucchini, tomato, and basil. Repeat the layers. Spread the remaining olive tapenade on the onion roll top, and place on top of the sandwich.

PER SERVING: *600 calories, 21 g protein, 41 g carbohydrates (9 g fiber), 40 g fat*

⫸ **PROTEIN BOOST**

Eat with Charred Green Beans with Roasted and Hot Peppers on page 162.

VEGGIE GRILLING 101

Preheat your grill to medium, and brush the sliced eggplant, yellow squash, and zucchini with olive oil. Add the veggie slices to the grill, then close the lid and cook until tender, about 10 minutes, flipping once halfway through.

Feta and Peas Sandwich

SERVES 1

WHAT YOU'LL NEED:

2 SLICES SOURDOUGH BREAD

1 GARLIC CLOVE

⅔ CUP SWEET PEAS, THAWED

1 TSP LEMON JUICE

½ TSP LEMON ZEST

2 TBSP CRUMBLED FETA

FRESH DILL SPRIGS

OLIVE OIL

1. Toast bread then rub one side of each slice with garlic.

2. In a bowl, mash peas with a fork and add lemon juice, lemon zest, and salt and pepper to taste.

3. Spread the pea mixture on one slice of bread and top with feta, dill sprigs, and a drizzle of olive oil. Top with remaining slice of bread.

PER SERVING: *560 calories, 23 g protein, 87 g carbohydrates (8 g fiber), 14 g fat*

||→ **PROTEIN BOOST**

Munch on Wasabi Peanuts on page 210, with this sandwich.

DON'T PASS ON PEAS

Peas are one of the easiest ways to add a fiber-and-vitamin turbo boost to your diet. They're packed with plant protein as well—eight grams in a one-cup serving.

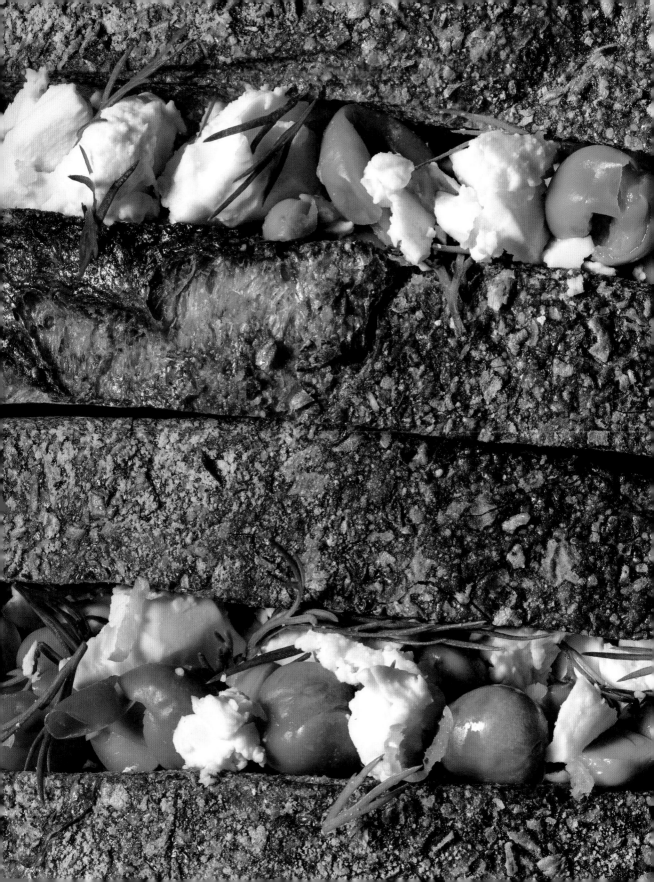

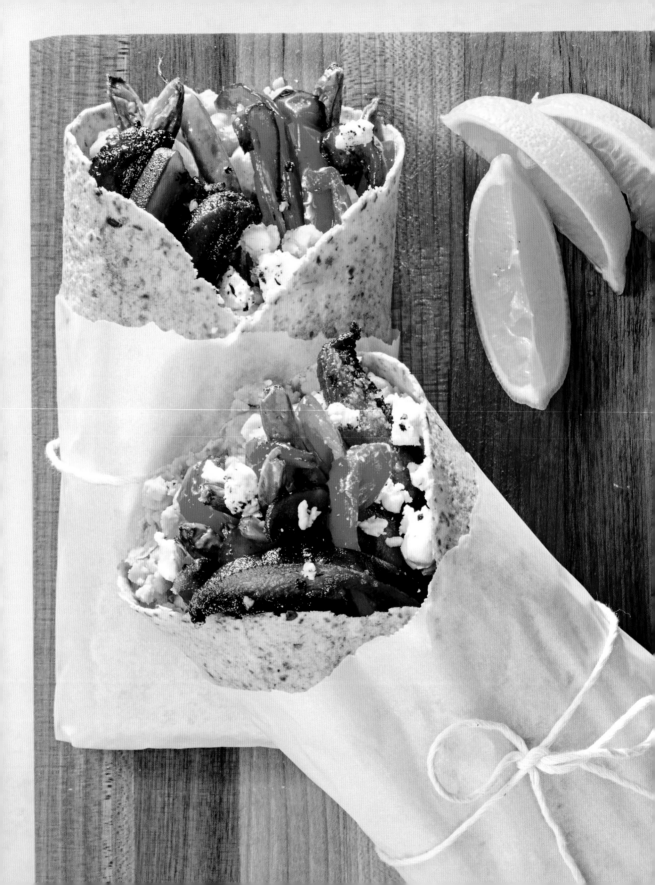

Vegetable Wraps with Goat Cheese

SERVES 4

WHAT YOU'LL NEED:

- 2 PORTOBELLO MUSHROOM CAPS, SLICED
- 1 LARGE RED BELL PEPPER, SLICED
- 8 OZ GREEN BEANS
- 2 TBSP OLIVE OIL
- 2 (15 OZ) CANS CHICKPEAS, DRAINED AND RINSED
- 3 TBSP LEMON JUICE
- 4 WHOLE-GRAIN WRAPS
- 1 OZ FRESH GOAT CHEESE, CRUMBLED
- LEMON WEDGES, FOR SERVING

1. Preheat your oven to 450°F. On two rimmed baking sheets, toss mushroom caps, red pepper, and green beans with olive oil and ¼ teaspoon salt. Roast until tender, 30 minutes.

2. Mash chickpeas with lemon juice and ¼ teaspoon pepper, then spread on wraps. Top with mushrooms, vegetables, and goat cheese. Wrap and serve with lemon wedges.

PER SERVING: *465 calories, 19 g protein, 66 g carbohydrates (17 g fiber), 6 g fat*

⫘→ **PROTEIN BOOST**

Grab a handful of Chickpea "Nuts" on page 205.

SHROOMS FOR IMPROVEMENT

Mushrooms are rich in ergothioneine, an amino acid that acts as an antioxidant that protects cells from abnormal growth and replication. In short, the antioxidant may reduce cancer risks; and researchers are looking into whether it might also reduce lung inflammation as well as liver, kidneys, and brain damage.

Grilled Greek Salad Pitas

SERVES 4

WHAT YOU'LL NEED:

- 4 WHOLE-WHEAT POCKET PITAS
- 8 OZ BLOCK COTIJA CHEESE, HALVED LENGTHWISE
- ½ CUP CHERRY TOMATOES, HALVED
- ½ ROMAINE HEART, CHOPPED
- ¼ CUP VERY THINLY SLICED RED ONION
- ¼ CUP PITTED KALAMATA OLIVES
- ½ CUCUMBER, PEELED, SEEDED, AND DICED
- LEAVES FROM 2 STEMS OREGANO, ROUGHLY CHOPPED
- 1 TSP OLIVE OIL

1. Preheat your oven to 200°F. In a large, dry cast-iron grill pan over medium-high, toast the pitas until grill marks appear, about 2 minutes on each side. Wrap the grilled pitas in foil and keep warm in the oven.

2. In the same grill pan over medium-high, add the cheese. Grill until marks appear, 2 to 4 minutes on each side. Transfer the cheese to a cutting board and roughly chop.

3. Add the tomatoes to the pan and cook until just blistered, about 2 minutes.

4. In a large bowl, toss everything except the pitas with the olive oil. Season to taste with salt and pepper. Slice the pitas in half. Stuff the mixture into the pita pockets.

PER SERVING: *446 calories, 30 g protein, 31 g carbohydrates (5 g fiber), 25 g fat*

GRILLED CHEESE

Cotija is a dry, crumbly Mexican cheese—the kind you get on street tacos. It doesn't melt particularly well, which is a good thing when it's being grilled.

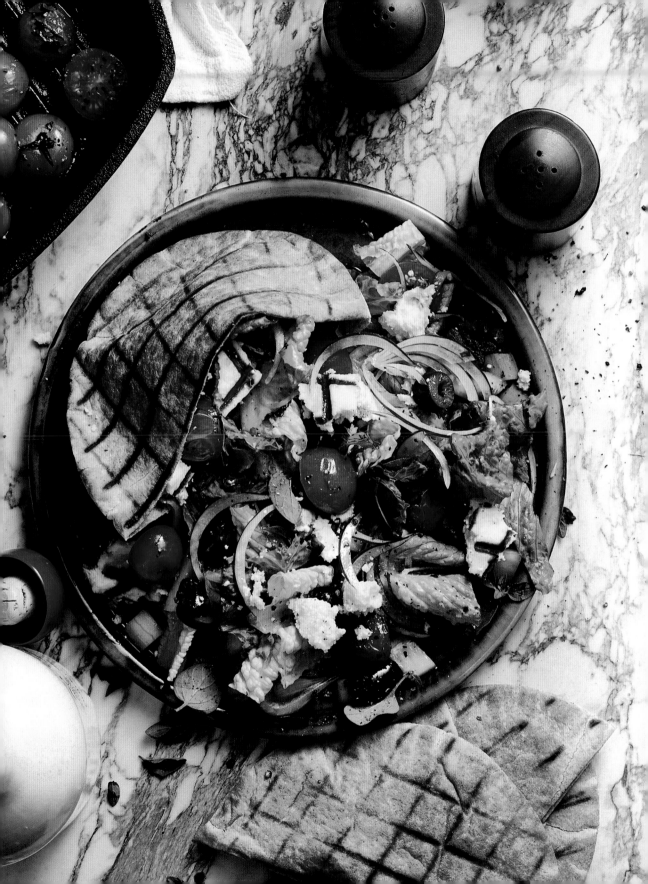

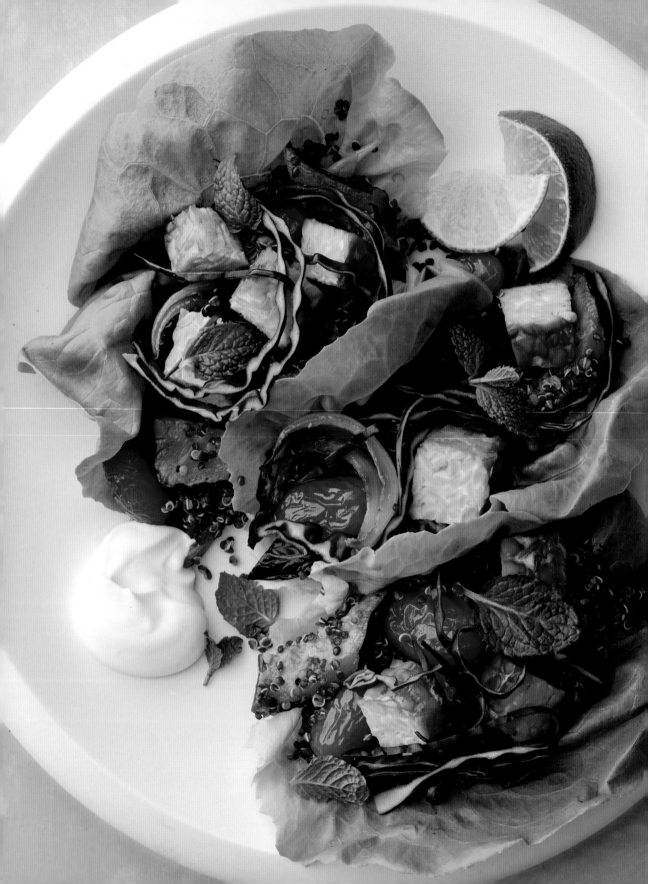

Tempeh Lettuce Wraps

SERVES 1

WHAT YOU'LL NEED:

- ½ CUP COOKED QUINOA
- ¼ CUP CHOPPED ZUCCHINI
- ¼ CUP CHOPPED ONION
- ¼ CUP CHOPPED TOMATO
- 3 BIBB LETTUCE LEAVES
- 1 PIECE ROASTED TEMPEH, CHOPPED
- ¼ CUP SHREDDED RED CABBAGE
- FRESH CILANTRO OR MINT
- 2 TBSP PLAIN GREEK YOGURT
- LIME WEDGES, FOR SERVING

1. In a bowl, combine the quinoa, zucchini, onion, and tomato. Season with a pinch each of coarse salt and pepper.

2. Spoon quinoa-vegetable mixture onto lettuce leaves, and top with tempeh, red cabbage, cilantro, and yogurt. Serve with lime wedges.

PER SERVING: *338 calories, 25 g protein, 42 g carbohydrates (12 g fiber), 10 g fat*

DON'T BE BITTER

Quinoa has a natural coating called saponin that can make it taste bitter or soapy. Most boxed quinoa doesn't have this coating, but you can't hurt the grain by giving it a good rinse under some cool water in a fine-mesh strainer before cooking.

Six Plant-Based Power Foods

A strong diet isn't just about protein. It's about choosing minimally processed foods with nutritional oomph. Here's a handful to add to your cart, if you're not already doing so.

THREE WAYS TO SHOP SMARTER

Ignore packaging billboards. The front of a food package is real estate owned by the processor whose goal is to sell you something. Flip the package over to find the nutrient information you need.

Shop outside. For the most part, stick to the perimeter of the store, where fresh produce, healthy carbs and fats, lean protein, and dairy hang out. Head to the interior aisles for ingredients such as canned beans and whole grains.

Double the value. If you think healthy food costs more than junk food, think again. Do a little planning—check out what's on sale and stock up. Buy produce in season to maximize quality, flavor, and cost.

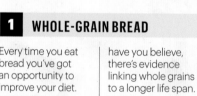

1 WHOLE-GRAIN BREAD

Every time you eat bread you've got an opportunity to improve your diet.

▶ **WHY IT'S GOOD:** Contrary to what carb haters would have you believe, there's evidence linking whole grains to a longer life span.

▶ **HOW TO EAT MORE:** For a smart snack, toast or grill one slice of bread and top it with a heaping helping of halved cherry tomatoes, marinated mushrooms, or avocado with sliced radishes.

2 LENTILS

These little UFO-shaped "pulses" are the edible seeds of legumes.

▶ **WHY IT'S GOOD:** Lentils are a plentiful source of fiber, protein, and essential nutrients (iron, manganese, and potassium), and a key source of riboflavin, magnesium, and zinc.

▶ **HOW TO EAT MORE:** Deploy them as a fortifier to burgers or meatballs. All lentil varieties have a mild, nutty flavor. Red and yellow types develop a softer texture when cooked, so save those for slow-simmered dishes. Brown and black lentils retain their texture better, which means they work best in heartier meals.

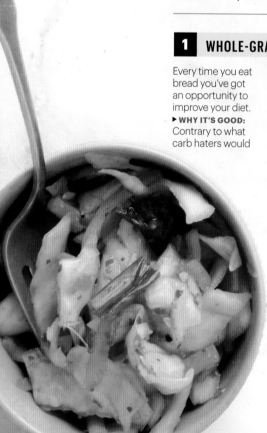

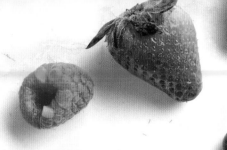
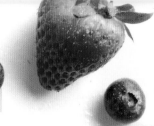
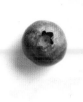
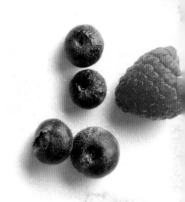
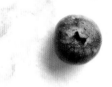

3 BEETS

Commonly blood red, beets also come in candy-cane and golden varieties. They're subtly sweet and hearty.

▸ **WHY IT'S GOOD:**
Many nutrients, few calories. Beets contain a bit of almost all of the vitamins and minerals that you need, plus inorganic nitrates and pigments that may enhance athletic performance if consumed 2 to 3 hours before training.

▸ **HOW TO EAT MORE:**
Roasted beets are great with a little olive oil, salt, and pepper as a simple side or addition to a salad or bowl. One downside, they can make your kitchen look like a crime scene. An option is to buy packaged, precooked beets. Or try pickled beets or golden beets to avoid the mess. (The golden variety has beneficial compounds like its red brethren.)

4 WATERCRESS

If leafy greens were the 2017 Philadelphia Eagles, watercress would be Nick Foles. It may not have as many believers as kale or spinach, but it'll deliver. Watercress has stubby, ear-shape leaves that top long, curved stems, and it tastes peppery.

▸ **WHY IT'S GOOD:**
Watercress is nutrient-dense, meaning it offers a large payload of nutrients per calorie.

▸ **HOW TO EAT MORE:**
Think of watercress as a zestier spinach. Chop a handful and stir it into frittatas, stir-fries, or marinara sauce for pasta. It's also delicious as a swap-in for basil in homemade pesto. You can enjoy it in a salad, but balance its bite with mellower greens like romaine, butter, or green leaf lettuce (like we did in the Beefy Salad, page 129).

5 KIMCHEE

Kimchee is a traditional Korean food made with cabbage, chile peppers, salt, and sometimes other vegetables, all of which undergo fermentation with lactic-acid bacteria. Its taste can range from mellow and tangy to pungent and spicy.

▸ **WHY IT'S GOOD:**
Your gastrointestinal tract, filled with billions of tiny microbes, may play a big role in your immune system and overall health. Good bacteria, called probiotics, may counterbalance disruptive bad bacteria. Found in foods like kimchee, probiotics may also help fight obesity, cholesterol, and cancer, though further research is needed.

▸ **HOW TO EAT MORE:**
Try kimchee in place of coleslaw, as a sandwich or taco topper, or scrambled into eggs. Aim to have 1 cup at least twice a week. Just make sure you buy kimchee unpasteurized—the kind found at a good supermarket or Korean grocery store. Pasteurization can kill probiotic bacteria.

6 BERRIES

Fresh or dried, strawberries, blueberries, blackberries, raspberries, and gooseberries are small-but-mighty nutritional powerhouses.

▸ **WHY THEY'RE GOOD:**
They are a great source of fiber (1 cup of fresh blueberries has almost 4 grams; 1 cup of blackberries has more than 7 grams), are high in antioxidants that help keep free radicals under control, improve blood sugar and insulin response, and are packed with vitamins and minerals.

▸ **HOW TO EAT MORE:**
Berries are delicious any time of day. Mix into a grain bowl, scatter over a salad, or nosh as a snack with a handful of nuts.

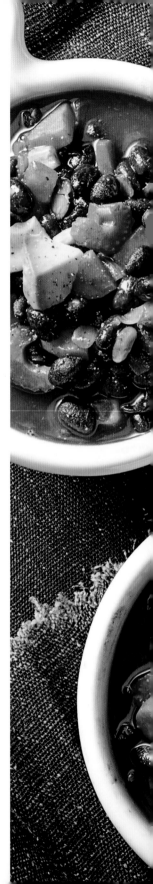

Salads & Soups

There's one big reason people think that soups and salads are boring: They're eating boring soups and salads. The recipes in this section will take you far beyond chicken noodle and chicken Caesar. They'll take you to magical lands of pure deliciousness.

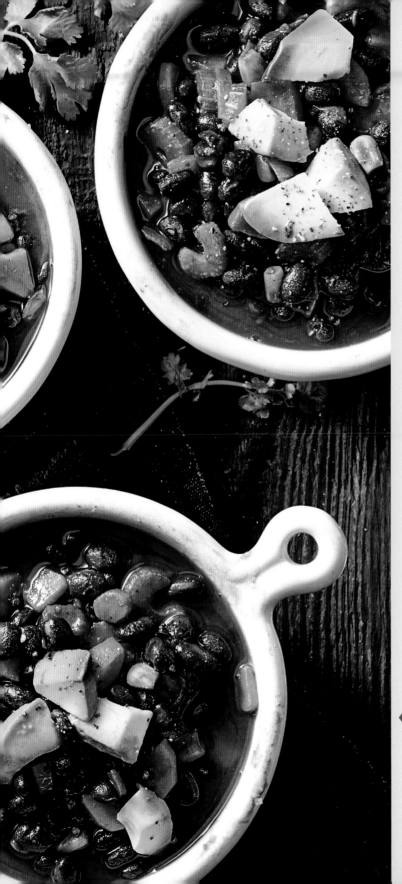

THE RECIPES

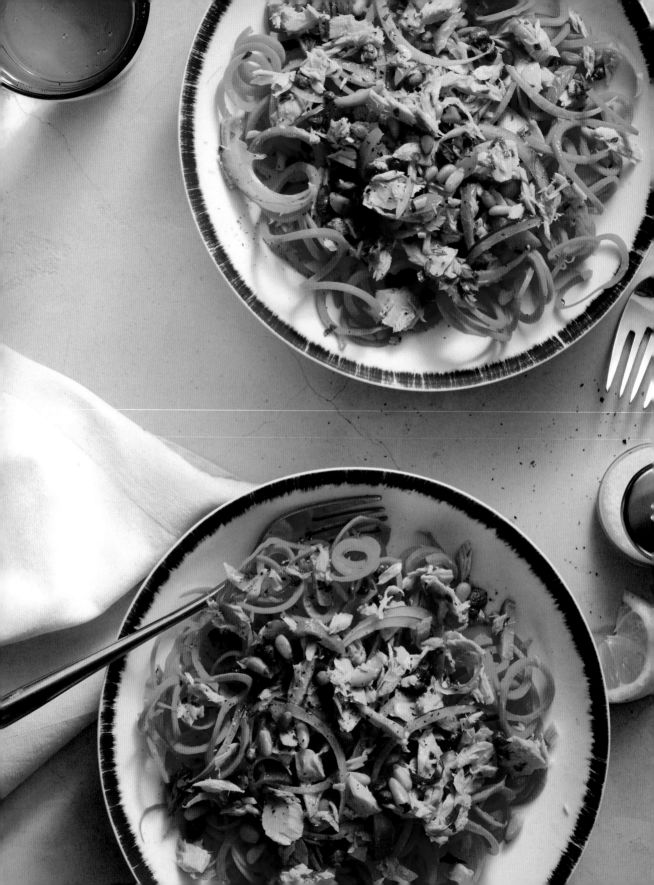

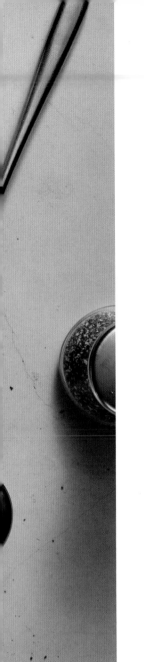

Carrot "Capellini" with Mediterranean Tuna Salad

SERVES 2

WHAT YOU'LL NEED

- 2 LARGE, THICK CARROTS, HALVED CROSSWISE
- 3 TBSP FRESH LEMON JUICE, DIVIDED (ABOUT 1½ LEMONS)
- 1 (4 OZ) CAN TUNA IN WATER, DRAINED
- 1½ CUP NAVY BEANS
- ½ SMALL RED ONION, THINLY SLICED
- ½ CUP FRESH FLAT-LEAF PARSLEY, CHOPPED
- ¼ CUP BRIGHT GREEN PITTED OLIVES, SLICED
- 2 TBSP PINE NUTS, TOASTED
- 1 TBSP CAPERS, RINSED
- 1 TBSP OLIVE OIL

1. Cut carrots on a vegetable spiral slicer using the smallest noodle attachment; transfer to a medium bowl and toss with 1 tablespoon of the lemon juice, ¼ teaspoon each salt and pepper.

2. In another bowl, gently toss the tuna, navy beans, onion, parsley, olives, pine nuts, capers, remaining 2 tablespoons lemon juice, and oil. Serve over carrot noodles.

PER SERVING: *489 calories, 25 g protein, 49 g carbohydrates (19 g fiber), 19 g fat*

GO GREENER

This recipe calls for green olives. You can use the pimento-stuffed Spanish Manzanilla olives you're used to, but bright-green Castelvetrano olives from Sicily also work really well. Castelvetrano olives are bright, buttery, and meaty.

Steak Salad with Greens, Peas, and Potatoes

SERVES 4

WHAT YOU'LL NEED:

- 2 TBSP RED WINE VINEGAR
- 1 TBSP DIJON MUSTARD
- 3 TBSP OLIVE OIL
- 12 OZ RED AND/OR YELLOW BABY POTATOES
- 1 (8 OZ) TOP SIRLOIN OR SIRLOIN TIP STEAK (ABOUT 1-INCH THICK)
- 1 TSP OLIVE OIL
- 6 CUPS PACKED BABY ARUGULA
- 1 TOMATO, CUT INTO WEDGES
- 2 LARGE BUTTON MUSHROOMS, THINLY SLICED
- ½ CUP FROZEN PEAS, THAWED

1. For the vinaigrette, combine the vinegar and mustard, and season with salt and pepper. Whisk in the oil.

2. Place a steamer basket in a saucepan of boiling water and steam potatoes until tender, about 20 minutes. Transfer to a bowl and let cool slightly. Using a spoon, lightly smash potatoes. Drizzle half of the vinaigrette over the potatoes.

3. Season steak on both sides with salt and pepper. In a cast-iron skillet (or other heavy skillet) over medium-high, heat the oil until almost smoking. Sear steak, about 8 minutes on each side for medium-rare. Transfer to a plate to rest a few minutes.

4. In a large bowl, toss the arugula with the remaining vinaigrette. Divide the arugula among 4 plates, and top with the smashed potatoes, tomato, mushrooms, and peas. Cut steak into ¼-inch slices and arrange on salads.

PER SERVING: *340 calories, 13 g protein, 21 g carbohydrates (3 g fiber), 22 g fat*

⫸ PROTEIN BOOST

For each salad, add ½ cup canned pinto beans, rinsed and drained, to meet your protein needs in one bowl. No additional dishes required.

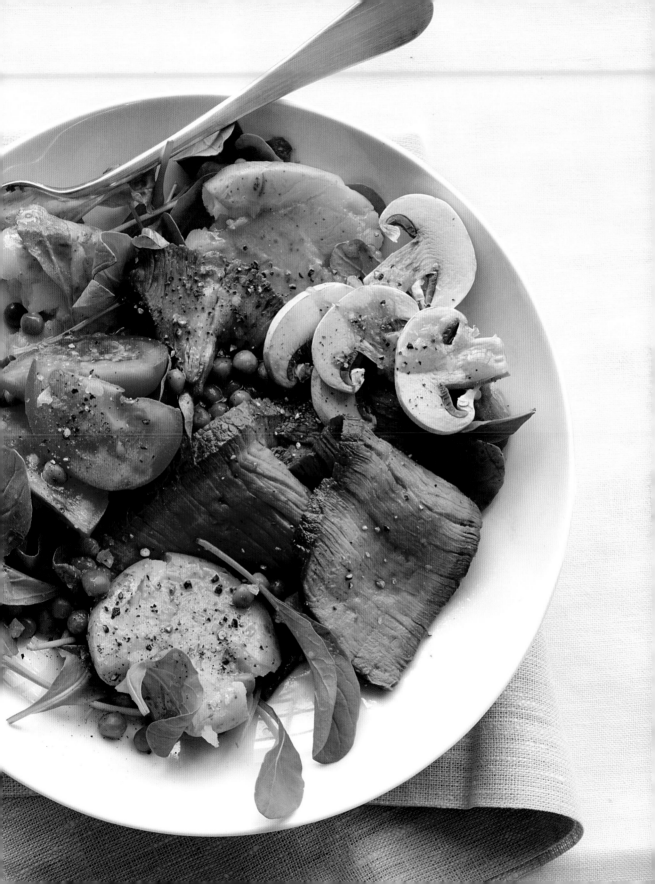

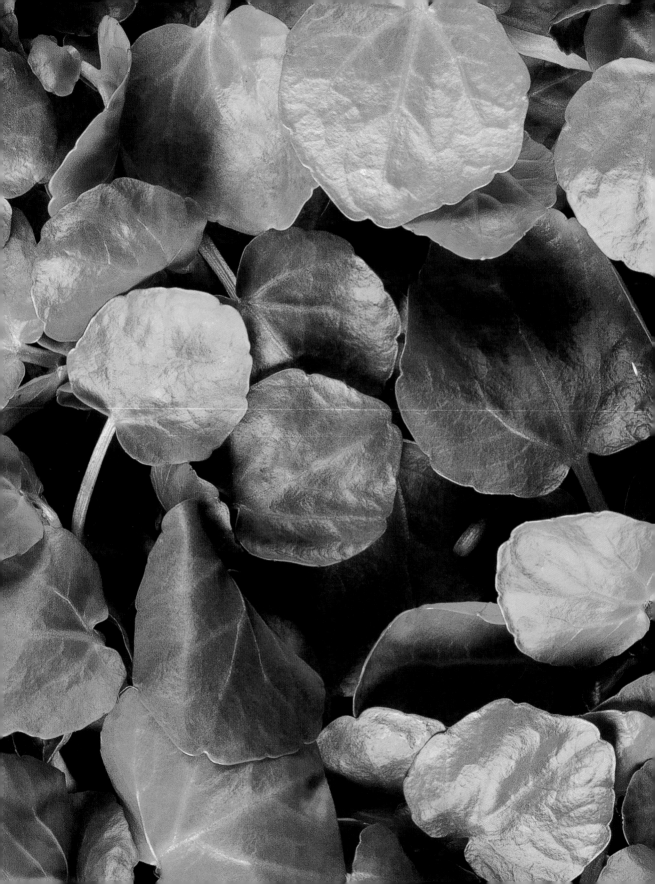

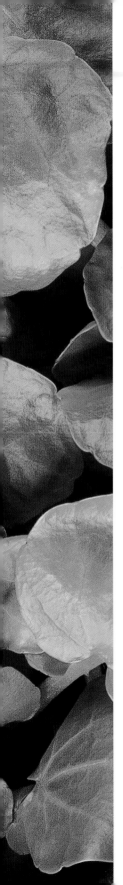

Beefy Salad

SERVES 1

WHAT YOU'LL NEED:

1 CUP CHOPPED ARUGULA

1 CUP CHOPPED ROMAINE

1 CUP CHOPPED WATERCRESS

½ CUP CHICKPEAS

¼ CUP ROASTED PUMPKIN SEEDS OR PEPITAS

¼ CUP ROASTED RED PEPPERS

2 TO 4 TBSP ITALIAN DRESSING

2 OZ LEFTOVER SIRLOIN STEAK, SLICED

1. In a large bowl, combine the arugula, romaine, and watercress. Add the chickpeas, pumpkin seeds, and red peppers. Drizzle with the Italian dressing and toss.

2. Transfer the salad to a plate and top with the sliced steak.

PER SERVING: *538 calories, 33 g protein, 33 g carbohydrates (10 g fiber), 32 g fat*

INCREDIBLE CRESS

This leafy green is a member of the cabbage family that grows in water. It adds a peppery kick to salads and sandwiches. One cup of watercress has just four calories, and it's loaded with vitamins A, C, and K. A study in the *American Journal of Clinical Nutrition* found that eating three ounces of watercress daily increased levels of the antioxidants lutein by 100 percent and beta-carotene by 33 percent, respectively. If you have trouble finding it, arugula makes a good substitute.

Bratwurst-Apple Salad with Caraway Vinaigrette

SERVES 4

WHAT YOU'LL NEED:

- 1 TSP CARAWAY SEEDS, CRUSHED
- 3 TBSP SHERRY VINEGAR
- 1 TBSP WHOLE-GRAIN MUSTARD
- ½ SMALL RED ONION, FINELY CHOPPED
- 4 VEGAN BRATWURSTS (ABOUT 12 OZ)
- 2 TBSP OLIVE OIL
- 1 SMALL FENNEL BULB, CORED AND THINLY SLICED
- 1 GALA APPLE, THINLY SLICED
- 6 CUPS MIXED GREENS

1. Heat a small pan over medium; add caraway seeds and toast until fragrant, about 2 minutes. In a large bowl, whisk together vinegar, mustard, ⅛ teaspoon each kosher salt and pepper. Mix in the caraway seeds and onion; let sit 5 minutes.

2. Meanwhile, cook bratwursts according to package instructions, then slice.

3. Toss onion mixture with oil, then fennel and apple. Fold in greens and bratwursts.

PER SERVING: *334 calories, 20 g protein, 19 g carbohydrates (7 g fiber), 21 g fat*

||→ **PROTEIN BOOST**

Scatter a handful of walnuts over this salad just before serving to add crunch and reach your protein goal.

START WITH SAUSAGE

If you're a dedicated meat eater looking to reform your diet with plant-based alternatives that won't make you miss the real thing, vegan sausage is a great place to start. First, there's the satisfying "snap" of the casing on pork sausage. The casing on most vegan sausage is made from alginate, which is a natural, 100% plant-based product derived from algae. It's actually used in some turkey and seafood sausages to deliver that same pop as animal casing.

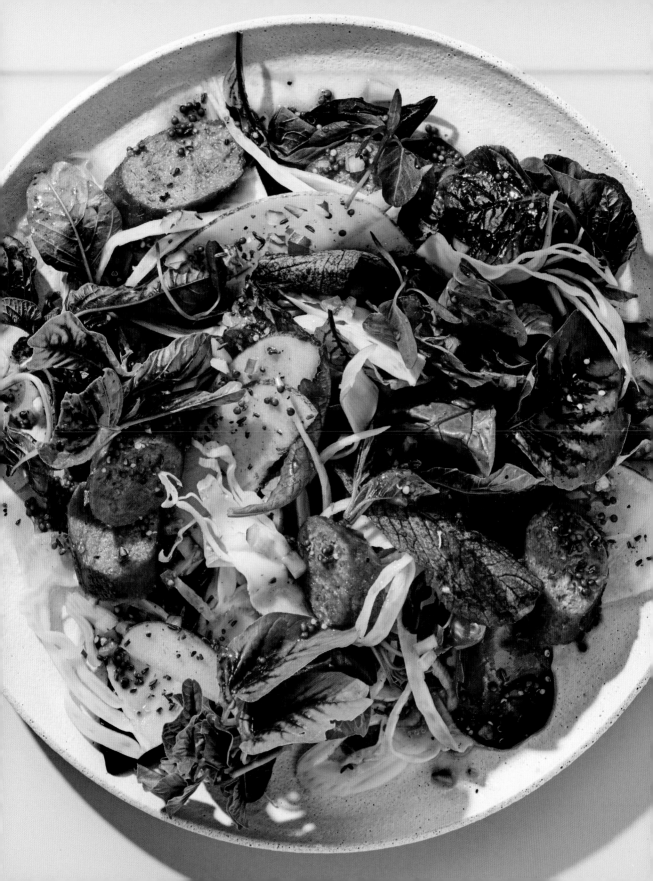

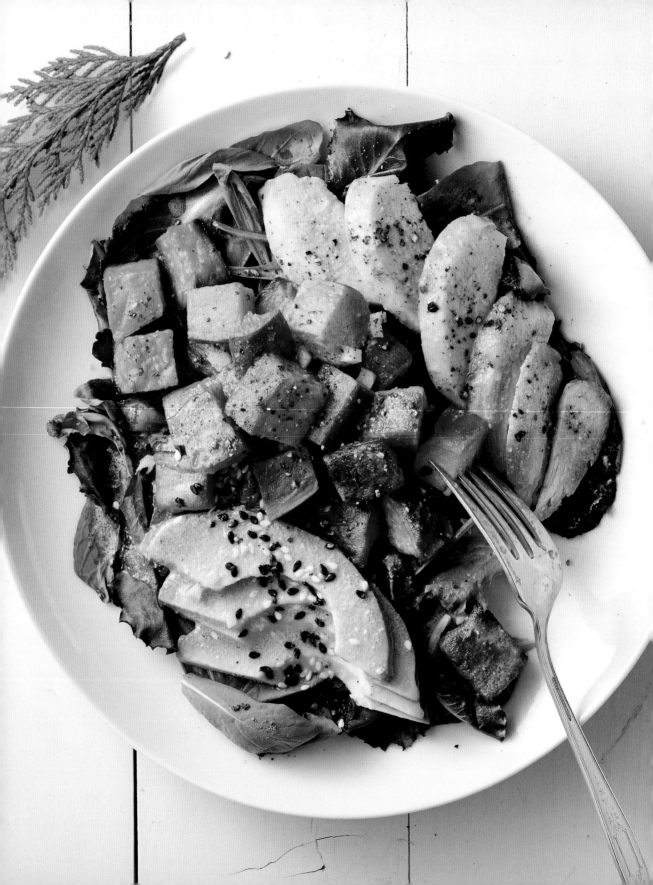

Roasted Sweet Potato and Chicken Salad

SERVES 4

WHAT YOU'LL NEED:

2½ LB SWEET POTATOES, CUT INTO ½-INCH CHUNKS

2 TBSP OLIVE OIL

¼ CUP SEASONED RICE VINEGAR

2 TBSP TOASTED SESAME OIL

1 TBSP MISO PASTE

1 TBSP FINELY CHOPPED PEELED FRESH GINGER

1 (20 OZ) BAG MIXED GREENS

2 ROTISSERIE CHICKEN BREAST HALVES (ABOUT 8 OZ), SLICED

1 AVOCADO, PITTED PEELED, AND SLICED

SESAME SEEDS, FOR SERVING

1. Preheat your oven to 450°F. On a large rimmed baking sheet, toss the sweet potatoes with oil and ¼ teaspoon salt; roast until tender, 25 minutes.

2. In a small bowl, whisk together rice vinegar, sesame oil, miso, ginger, and ¼ teaspoon pepper.

3. Divide mixed greens, sweet potatoes, chicken, and avocado among 4 plates. Drizzle with miso vinaigrette and top with sesame seeds.

PER SERVING: *517 calories, 25 g protein, 54 g carbohydrates (14 g fiber), 24 g fat*

KNOW YOUR MISO

Like other soy-based foods, miso is a good source of antioxidant minerals like copper, manganese, and zinc. There are three types of miso—white, which has a mild, slightly sweet flavor; yellow, which is fermented longer than white and has a slightly more intense flavor; and red, which has a rich, mature umami flavor. Choose whichever you like best.

Hearty Kale and Bean Salad

SERVES 4

WHAT YOU'LL NEED:

10 OZ TUSCAN KALE

2 CUPS THINLY SLICED BRUSSELS SPROUTS

JUICE OF 1 LEMON

1 GARLIC CLOVE, MINCED

3 TBSP OLIVE OIL

1 (15 OZ) CAN CANNELLINI BEANS, RINSED AND DRAINED

⅓ CUP TOASTED WALNUTS

1 CUP GRATED PARMESAN

SOURDOUGH OR MULTIGRAIN BREAD, TOASTED, FOR SERVING (OPTIONAL)

1. In a large serving bowl, mix the kale and Brussels sprouts.

2. In a small bowl, whisk the lemon juice, garlic, ¼ teaspoon each salt and pepper. Whisk in oil.

3. Toss the dressing with the kale mixture. Add the cannellini beans, walnuts, and Parmesan, and toss again. If desired, serve with toasted bread.

PER SERVING: *455 calories, 25 g protein, 33 g carbohydrates (13 g fiber), 27 g fat*

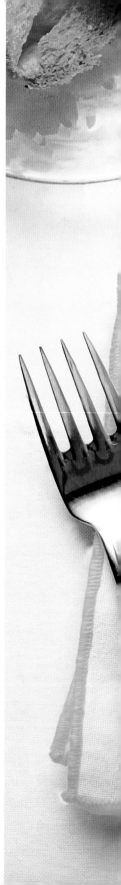

WARM YOUR NUTS

Toasting nuts intensifies their flavor. Here's how you do it: In a dry pan over medium heat add the nuts and toast, shaking the pan every now and then, until aromatic. Depending on the nut and the heat of your stovetop, this can take three to seven minutes.

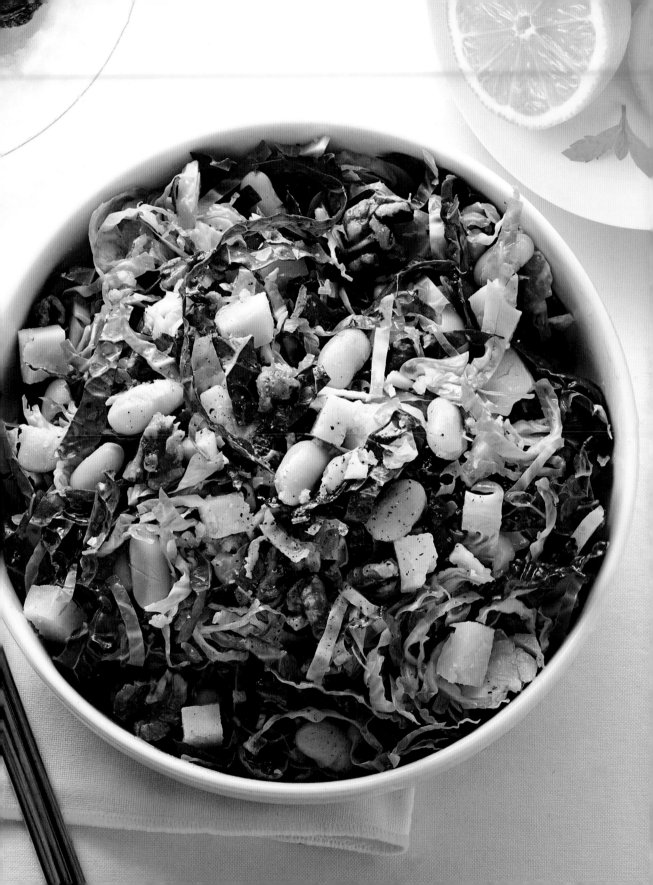

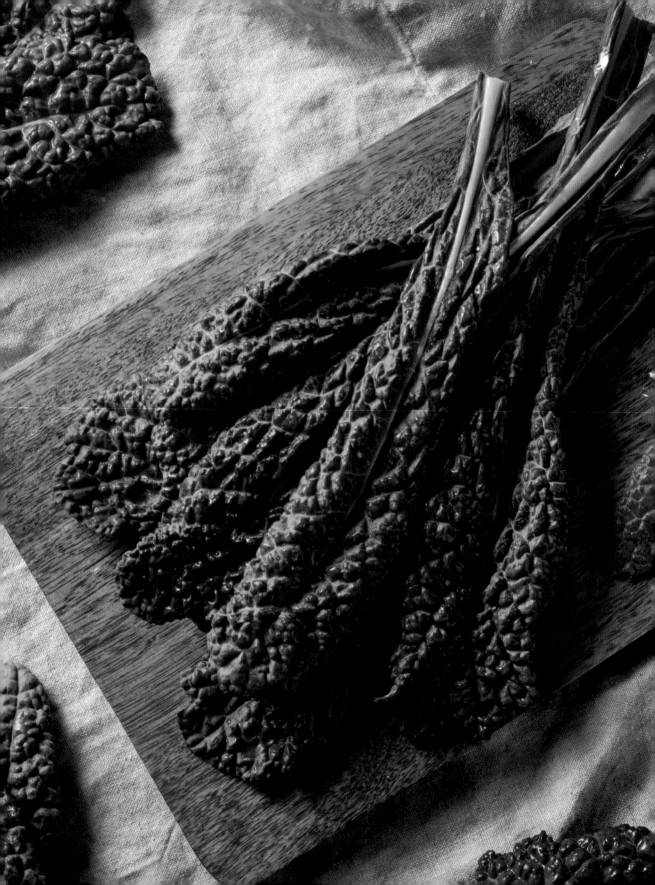

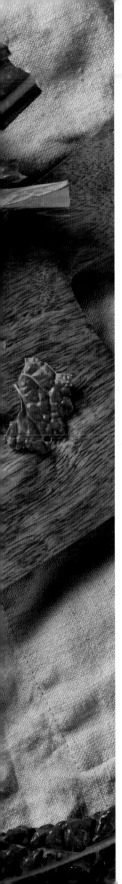

BBQ Kale Salad

SERVES 1

WHAT YOU'LL NEED:

- 2 CUPS CHOPPED DINOSAUR KALE
- ¼ CUP BARBECUE PULLED PORK
- ¾ CUP BLACK BEANS
- ¼ CUP FROZEN CORN, THAWED
- ¼ CUP CHOPPED ROASTED RED PEPPERS
- ½ AVOCADO, PITTED, PEELED, AND SLICED
- 4 TBSP PACKAGED SOUTHWEST-STYLE DRESSING

Arrange the kale on a plate, and add the pork, black beans, corn, roasted red peppers, and sliced avocado. Drizzle with the dressing.

PER SERVING: *786 calories, 26 g protein, 80 g carbohydrates (23 g fiber), 44 g fat*

KALE YEAH!

The most familiar kale is the curly-leaf kind, but that's not all that's out there. Dinosaur kale (also called Tuscan or Lacinato kale) is named for its nubby texture. It has a milder flavor and more tender texture than the curly-leaf stuff. Whatever type you choose, kale is almost unsurpassed in its nutrient density. It's rich in vitamins A, C, and K, potassium, calcium, iron, and folate, as well as the eye-healthy carotenoids lutein and zeaxanthin.

Seared Scallops and Lentil Salad

SERVES 4

WHAT YOU'LL NEED:

- 1¼ CUPS GREEN FRENCH LENTILS
- 1 BUNCH KALE, RIBS REMOVED, THINLY SLICED
- 2½ CUPS SHREDDED CARROTS
- ¼ CUP BALSAMIC VINEGAR
- 1 TBSP DIJON MUSTARD
- 2 TBSP CANOLA OIL
- 12 SCALLOPS (ABOUT ¾ LB)
- CHOPPED FRESH CHIVES

1. Cook the lentils according to package instructions. Drain. While the lentils are still hot, toss with the kale, carrots, vinegar, mustard, and ½ teaspoon each salt and pepper.

2. In an extra-large skillet, heat the canola oil on medium-high until almost smoking. Pat any moisture from scallops with paper towels. Season with ½ teaspoon each salt and pepper. Cook scallops until well-browned on the bottom; flip and cook until well-browned on the bottom and no longer translucent, about 2 minutes per side.

3. Serve scallops over lentil salad and top with chives.

PER SERVING: *360 calories, 31 g protein, 51 g carbohydrates (11 g fiber), 5 g fat*

LENTILS: THE UNDERRATED LEGUME

French lentils are smaller than green lentils. They also have an earthy, peppery flavor and a firmer texture. They hold their shape well when cooked, which makes them great for salads, but they can also be used in brothy soups and side dishes. Their thicker skin means they take a little longer to cook than green lentils— usually 40 to 45 minutes. You can also buy them precooked to save some time.

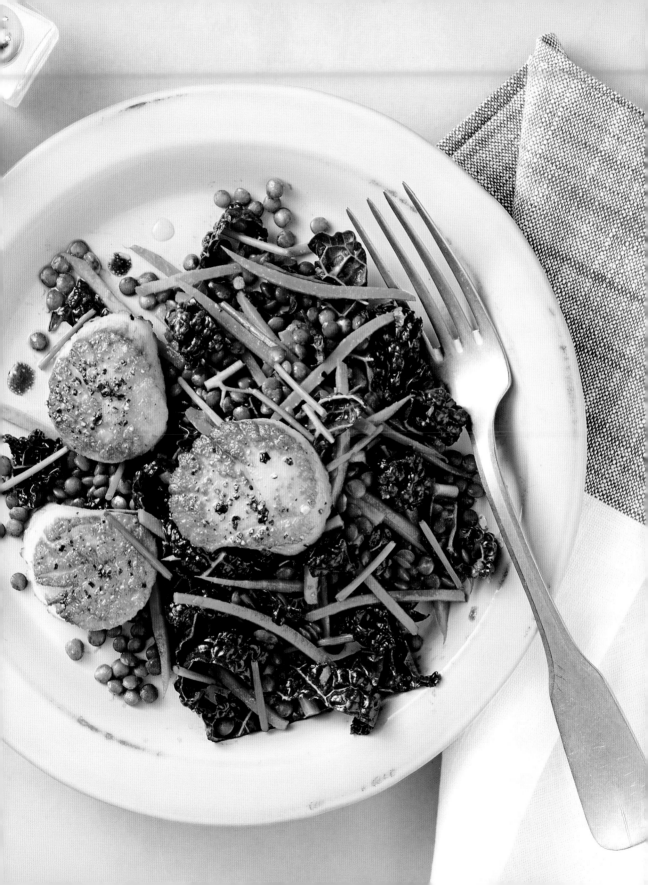

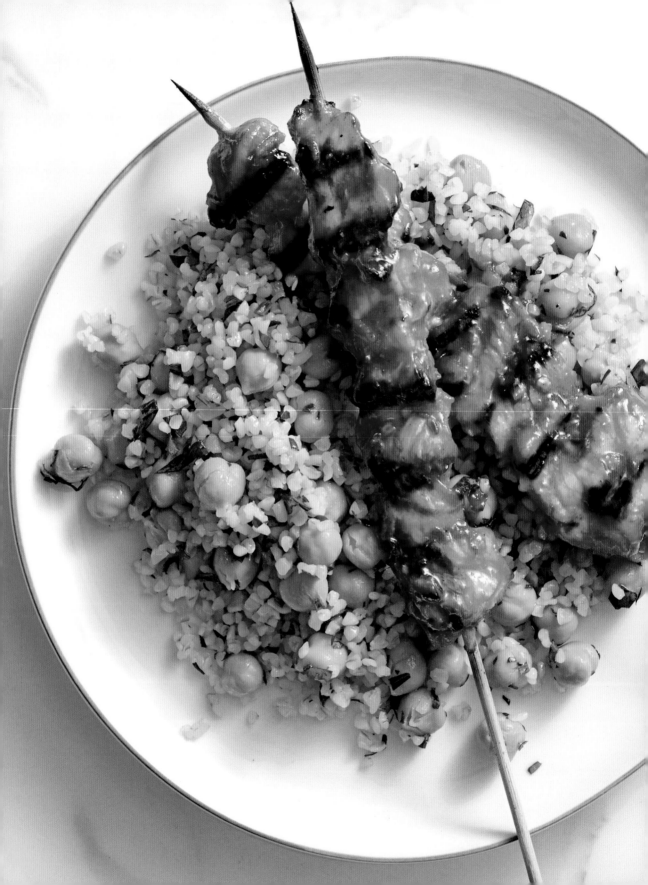

Harissa Grilled Chicken Kabob with Chickpea Bulgur Salad

SERVES 4

WHAT YOU'LL NEED:

- ¼ CUP HARISSA PEPPER PASTE
- 2 TBSP OLIVE OIL
- 2 TBSP HONEY
- 1½ CUPS DRY BULGUR
- 1 (19 OZ) CAN CHICKPEAS, RINSED AND DRAINED
- ¾ CUP FINELY CHOPPED FRESH PARSLEY
- 8 OZ SKINLESS, BONELESS CHICKEN BREAST, THINLY SLICED

1. In a large bowl, whisk the harissa paste with olive oil and honey; set half aside for serving.

2. In a saucepan, combine the bulgur and 2 cups water. Bring to a boil over medium-high, then reduce to a simmer. Cook, covered, until tender, about 12 minutes. Drain any excess liquid. Fluff bulgur with a fork. Add chickpeas, parsley, and ½ teaspoon salt to bulgur. Cover to keep warm.

3. Toss chicken with the remaining harissa mixture, then thread slices onto skewers. Preheat your grill to medium-high. Lightly oil the grill grates. Grill, turning once, until cooked through, 6 minutes.

4. Serve chicken on salad with reserved harissa sauce.

PER SERVING: *443 calories, 25 g protein, 64 g carbohydrates (14 g fiber), 12 g fat*

HAIL HARISSA

Harissa—a fiery pepper paste—pops up in North African, Middle Eastern, and Mediterranean cuisines. Its flavor comes from hot peppers, garlic, and spices. A cross between a paste and a sauce, harissa blends easily into curries and stews. You can also serve it alongside or on top of any dish that needs heat and tang. Find harissa in the grocery store (try Mina or Mediterranean Gourmet brands).

Soba Salad

SERVES 2

WHAT YOU'LL NEED:

- ½ CUP HUMMUS
- ¼ CUP SEASONED RICE VINEGAR
- 2 TBSP CANOLA OIL
- 1 TBSP SOY SAUCE
- 8 OZ SOBA NOODLES, COOKED
- 1 CUP FROZEN SHELLED EDAMAME, THAWED
- 1 CUP SHREDDED RED CABBAGE
- ½ CUP ROASTED CASHEWS
- BLACK OR WHITE SESAME SEEDS

1. In a bowl, whisk the hummus, rice vinegar, canola oil, soy sauce, and ¼ teaspoon salt.

2. Toss the hummus mixture with the soba noodles, edamame, cabbage, and cashews. Top servings with sesame seeds.

PER SERVING: *512 calories, 20 g protein, 69 g carbohydrates (4 g fiber), 21 g fat*

PROTEIN BOOST

Add 4 ounces stir-fried tofu with the edamame in Step 2.

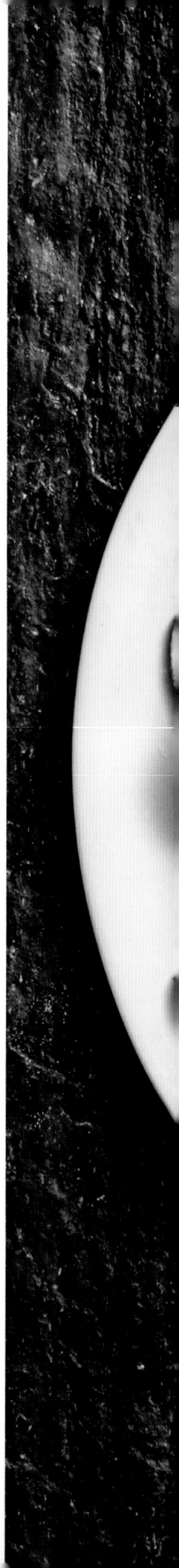

SOBA: SO GOOD

Japanese soba noodles are made from either all buckwheat flour or a blend of buckwheat and wheat flours. They're higher in fiber and protein than many other noodles and have a nutty, earthy flavor.

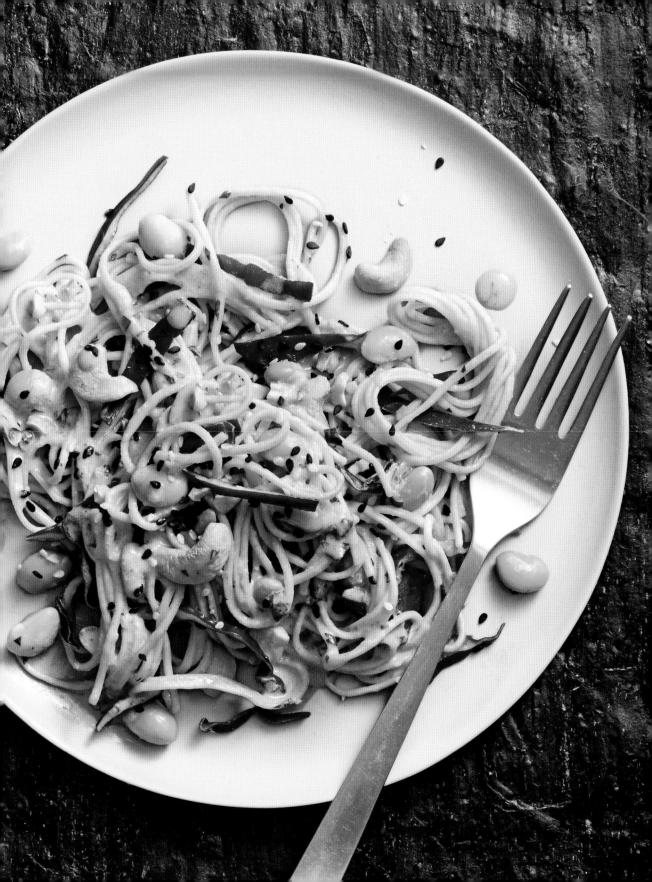

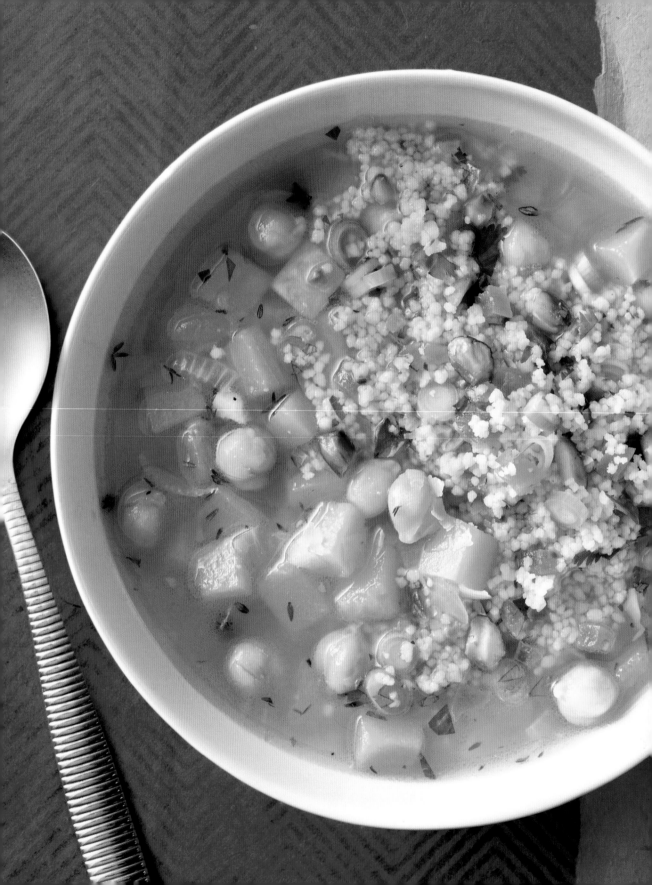

Butternut Squash and White Bean Soup

SERVES 4

WHAT YOU'LL NEED:

- 2 TBSP OLIVE OIL, DIVIDED
- 2 CUPS DICED BUTTERNUT SQUASH
- 1 MEDIUM ONION, CHOPPED
- 2 GARLIC CLOVES, MINCED
- 1 TBSP PEELED FRESH GINGER, FINELY CHOPPED
- 6 CUPS LOW-SODIUM CHICKEN BROTH
- 6 SPRIGS FRESH THYME
- 1 (15 OZ) CAN WHITE BEANS, RINSED AND DRAINED
- 1 (15 OZ) CAN CHICKPEAS, RINSED AND DRAINED
- ½ CUP WHOLE-GRAIN COUSCOUS
- ¼ CUP ROASTED PISTACHIOS, CHOPPED
- ¼ CUP FINELY CHOPPED DRIED APRICOTS
- ¼ CUP CHOPPED FRESH CILANTRO
- 1 SCALLION, SLICED

1. In a large skillet over medium, heat 1 tablespoon olive oil. Add the squash and cook, covered, stirring occasionally, until tender, 8 minutes.

2. Meanwhile, in a large pot over medium, heat the remaining 1 tablespoon oil. Add the onion and cook, covered, stirring occasionally, until tender, 6 minutes. Stir in the garlic and ginger and cook 1 minute.

3. Add the broth, thyme, and butternut squash to the pot and bring to a boil. Using a fork, mash the white beans and add to the soup along with the chickpeas. Season with salt and pepper to taste.

4. Cook the couscous according to package instructions and fluff with a fork. Fold in the pistachios, apricots, cilantro, and scallion. Serve the soup topped with the couscous mixture.

PER SERVING: *560 calories, 26 g protein, 88 g carbohydrates (19 g fiber), 16 g fat,*

Winter Squash and Lentil Stew

SERVES 4

WHAT YOU'LL NEED:

- 1 TBSP OLIVE OIL
- 2 MEDIUM SHALLOTS, THINLY SLICED
- 1 TBSP FINELY CHOPPED PEELED FRESH GINGER
- 1 TSP GROUND CORIANDER
- ½ TSP GROUND CARDAMOM
- 1 SMALL BUTTERNUT SQUASH, PEELED, SEEDED, AND CUT INTO 1½-INCH CHUNKS
- 1 LB GREEN LENTILS
- 6 CUPS CHICKEN OR VEGETABLE BROTH
- 5 CUPS PACKED BABY SPINACH
- 1 TBSP APPLE CIDER VINEGAR

1. In a large pot over medium, heat the oil. Cook shallots and ginger until shallots are golden, stirring frequently, 5 minutes. Add coriander and cardamom and cook 1 minute, stirring. Add squash, lentils, broth, and ¼ teaspoon salt.

2. Bring to a boil, then reduce heat and simmer, covered, until lentils are tender, 20 to 30 minutes.

3. Stir in spinach, vinegar, and ½ teaspoon each salt and pepper.

PER SERVING: *488 calories, 29 g protein, 86 g carbohydrates (23 g fiber), 6 g fat*

FOOD FOR THOUGHT

Butternut squash is a gold mine of beta-carotene—and Harvard researchers found that men who consumed more beta-carotene over 15 years had significantly delayed cognitive aging.

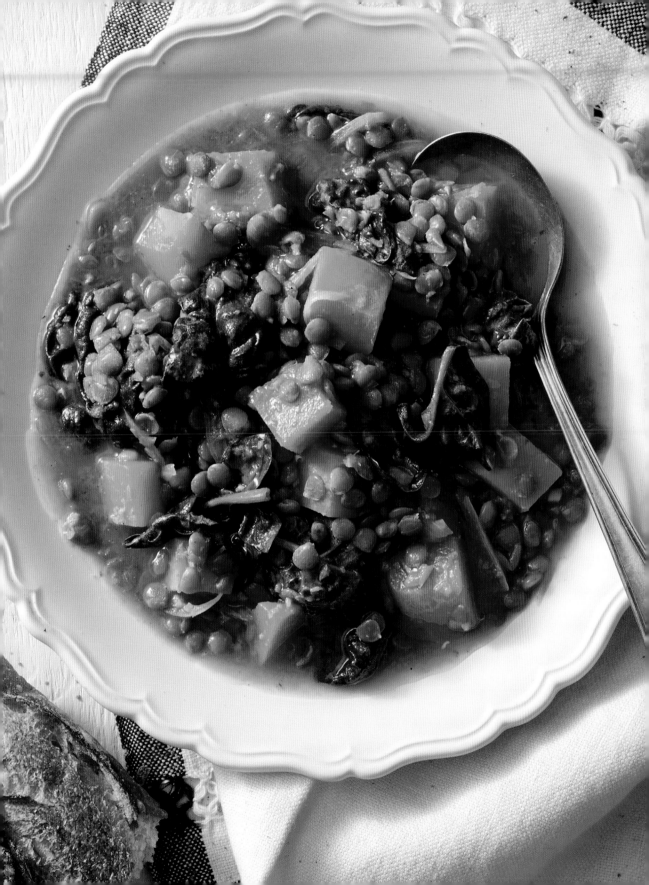

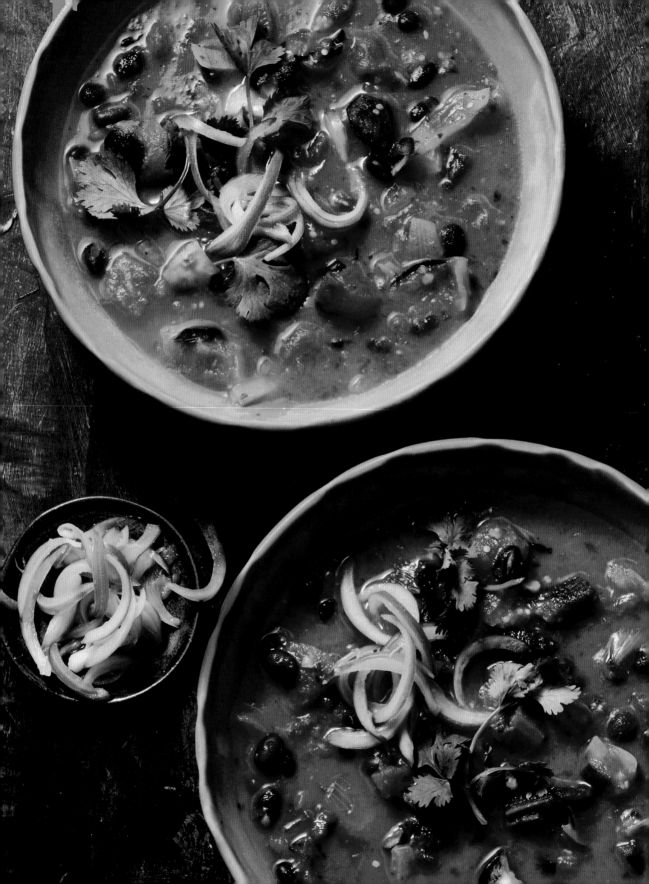

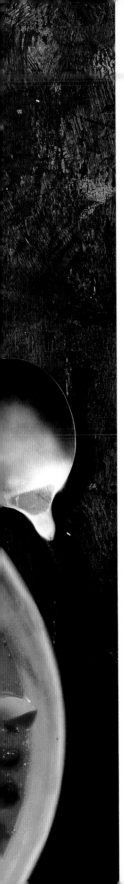

Fiery Black Bean Soup

SERVES 4

WHAT YOU'LL NEED:

8 OZ TOMATILLOS (ABOUT 4), HUSKED, RINSED WELL, AND HALVED

2 GARLIC CLOVES, UNPEELED

1 LARGE ONION, CUT INTO 1-INCH-THICK WEDGES

1 JALAPEÑO, HALVED AND SEEDED

1 TBSP OLIVE OIL

1 LARGE POBLANO PEPPER, HALVED AND SEEDED

½ TSP GROUND CUMIN

½ TSP GROUND CORIANDER

4 CUPS LOW-SODIUM CHICKEN BROTH

2 (15 OZ) CANS LOW-SODIUM BLACK BEANS, RINSED AND DRAINED

1 (14.5 OZ) CAN FIRE-ROASTED DICED TOMATOES, DRAINED

1 SMALL RED ONION, THINLY SLICED

2 TBSP FRESH LIME JUICE

FRESH CILANTRO LEAVES, FOR SERVING

1. Preheat your broiler. On a large rimmed baking sheet, toss tomatillos, garlic, onion wedges, jalapeños, oil, and a pinch each kosher salt and pepper. Add the poblano pepper, cut sides down, and broil, rotating pan every 5 minutes, until vegetables are tender and charred, about 15 minutes.

2. When cool enough to handle, discard skins from the poblano halves and garlic. Finely chop vegetables and transfer to a large pot. Add cumin and coriander and cook over medium, stirring occasionally, 2 minutes. Add broth, beans, and tomatoes, and bring to a simmer; cook 4 minutes.

3. Meanwhile, toss red onion with lime juice and a pinch each salt and pepper; let stand at least 10 minutes. Serve soup topped with pickled onion slices and cilantro.

PER SERVING: *325 calories, 20 g protein, 53 g carbohydrates (18 g fiber), 6 g fat*

||⊢→ **PROTEIN BOOST**

Top each serving with 2 tablespoons Greek yogurt and roasted pepitas.

Kale and Chickpea Soup

SERVES 4

WHAT YOU'LL NEED:

1 TBSP OLIVE OIL

6 GARLIC CLOVES, MINCED

ZEST FROM 1 LEMON

½ TSP FENNEL SEEDS, CRUSHED

¼ TSP CRUSHED RED PEPPER FLAKES

1 (4 OZ) CAN TOMATO PURÉE

1 BUNCH TUSCAN KALE, STEMS REMOVED AND COARSELY CHOPPED

1 (15.5 OZ) CAN CHICKPEAS, DRAINED AND RINSED

⅓ CUP GRATED PECORINO ROMANO CHEESE

LEMON WEDGES, FOR SERVING (OPTIONAL)

1. In a large pot over medium, heat the oil. Add garlic and lemon zest, and cook, stirring, 1 minute. Add fennel seeds and red pepper flakes, and cook, stirring, 2 minutes.

2. Add 4 cups water, tomato puree, and 1 teaspoon salt; cover and bring to a boil. Add kale and simmer until wilted, 4 minutes.

3. Add chickpeas and simmer until heated through, about 2 minutes. Serve with Pecorino Romano cheese and, if desired, lemon wedges.

PER SERVING: *335 calories, 20 g protein, 48 g carbohydrates (11 g fiber), 10 g fat*

⫸ PROTEIN BOOST

Stir in 1 cup plant-based meat crumbles with the chickpeas.

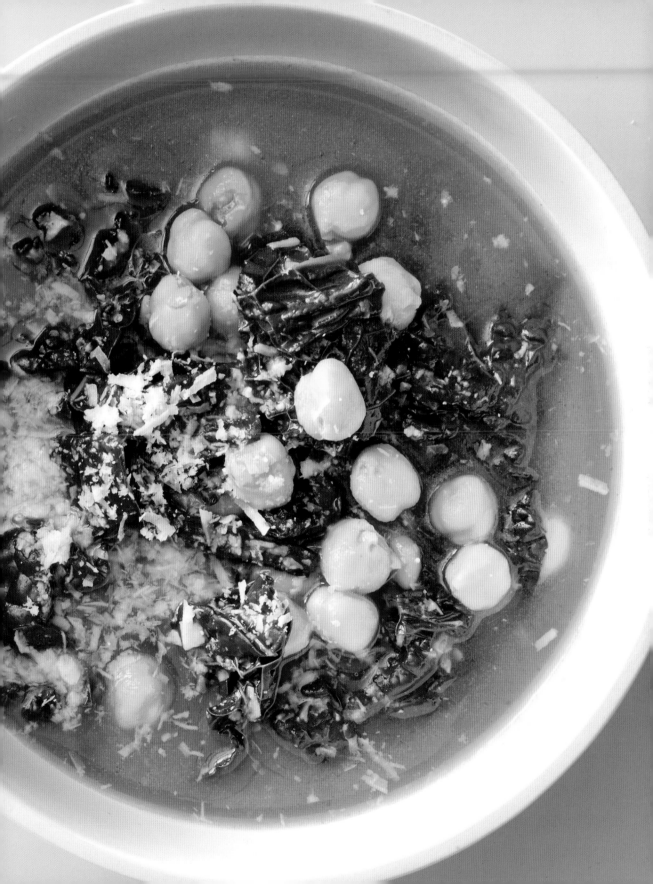

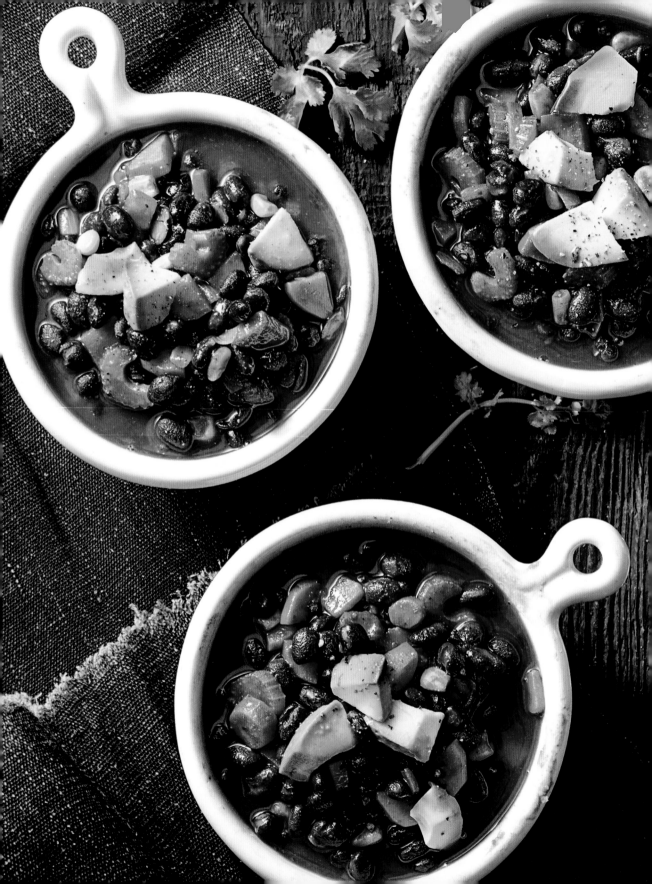

Smoky Black Bean Chili

SERVES 4

WHAT YOU'LL NEED:

- 2 TBSP OLIVE OIL
- 2 MEDIUM CARROTS, PEELED AND CHOPPED
- 2 STALKS CELERY, SLICED
- 1 MEDIUM ONION, FINELY CHOPPED
- ¼ CUP TOMATO PASTE
- 3 GARLIC CLOVES, MINCED
- 1½ TSP GROUND CUMIN
- 3 CUPS LOW-SODIUM VEGETABLE OR CHICKEN BROTH, DIVIDED
- 3 (15 OZ) CANS LOW-SODIUM BLACK BEANS, UNDRAINED
- 1 CUP FROZEN CORN
- DICED AVOCADO AND FRESH CILANTRO LEAVES, FOR SERVING

1. In a large pot over medium-high, heat the oil. Add the carrots, celery, and onion, and cook until starting to brown, stirring occasionally, 6 to 8 minutes. Add the tomato paste, garlic, and cumin, and cook, stirring, until the garlic is golden and the tomato paste has browned, 1 to 2 minutes. Stir in ½ cup broth, scraping up any browned bits on the bottom of the skillet.

2. Add the beans, corn, and remaining broth, and cook, covered, 30 to 45 minutes. Serve with avocado and cilantro and season with salt and pepper to taste.

PER SERVING: *489 calories, 21 g protein, 77 g carbohydrates (29 g fiber), 17 g fat*

⊩⟶ **PROTEIN BOOST**

Add protein to your meal with a couple of Date and Nut Energy Balls on page 214.

CHEW THE (GOOD) FAT

A staggering 77 percent of the calories in a single avocado are from fat. It's oleic acid, a monounsaturated fatty acid that is also found in olive oil. Oleic acid has a bunch of health benefits, which includes reducing disease-stoking inflammation.

Chipotle Lentil Chili

SERVES 4

WHAT YOU'LL NEED:

1 TBSP OLIVE OIL

1 MEDIUM ONION, CHOPPED

1 MEDIUM GREEN BELL PEPPER, CHOPPED

1 TBSP CHILI POWDER

2 CHIPOTLES IN ADOBO

2 GARLIC CLOVES

½ CUP SUN-DRIED TOMATOES

1 (28 OZ) CAN WHOLE PEELED TOMATOES, DRAINED

4 CUPS LOWER-SODIUM VEGETABLE BROTH

2 CUPS BROWN LENTILS

DICED AVOCADO, CHEDDAR CHEESE, FRESH CILANTRO LEAVES, AND TORTILLA CHIPS, FOR SERVING

1. In a large pot over medium, heat the olive oil. Add onion and pepper, and cook until softened, 3 minutes. Stir in chili powder, and cook 1 minute.

2. In a food processor, puree chipotles, garlic, and sun-dried tomatoes; pulse in whole peeled tomatoes until chopped. Add tomato mixture, broth, lentils, and ½ teaspoon salt to the pot.

3. Cook over medium, covered, until lentils are tender, 20 to 30 minutes. Serve with avocado, cheddar, cilantro, and tortilla chips.

PER SERVING: *465 calories, 29 g protein, 78 g carbohydrates (27 g fiber), 6 g fat*

CHILL YOUR CHILES

No matter how hot you like your food, you're probably never going to use an entire can of chipotle chiles in a single recipe. They're easily frozen for future use. Divide the remaining chiles and sauce in two-chile portions, and freeze in small containers or plastic bags for up to six months.

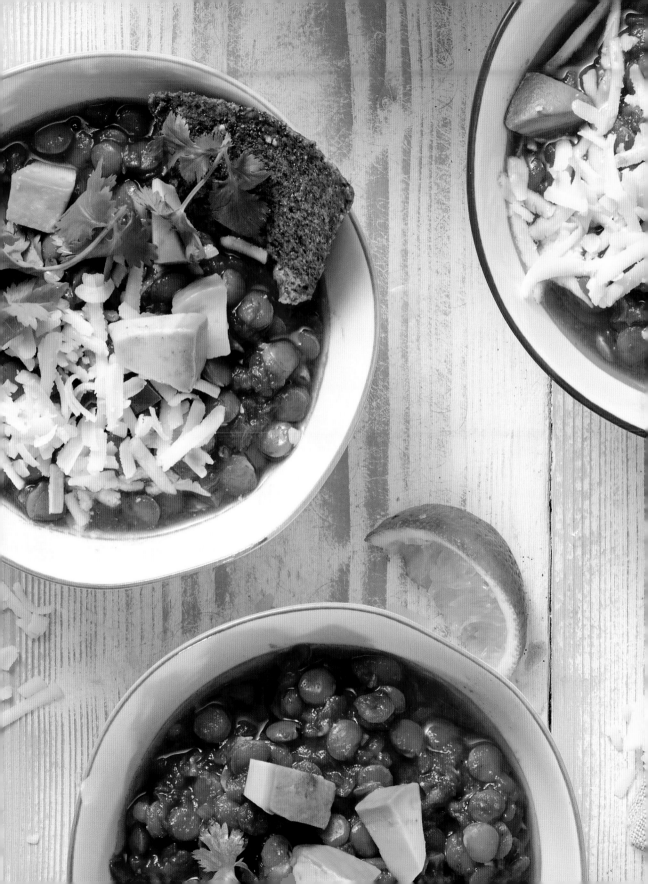

Tomato Soup
with Quinoa

SERVES 4

WHAT YOU'LL NEED:

2 TBSP OLIVE OIL + 1½ TSP, DIVIDED

1 LARGE ONION, COARSELY CHOPPED

2 LARGE GARLIC CLOVES, FINELY CHOPPED

1 TBSP CHOPPED FRESH THYME, PLUS MORE FOR SERVING

1 (28 OZ) CAN WHOLE PEELED PLUM TOMATOES, UNDRAINED

2½ CUPS LOW-SODIUM CHICKEN OR VEGETABLE BROTH

2 TBSP TOMATO PASTE

1½ CUPS COOKED QUINOA (FROM ABOUT ½ CUP UNCOOKED)

4 LARGE EGGS

HOT SAUCE, FOR SERVING

1. In a large saucepan over medium, heat 1 tablespoon oil. Add onion, garlic, thyme, and ½ teaspoon salt, and cook until onion is softened, about 3 minutes. Add tomatoes and their juice, broth, and tomato paste, and bring to a boil. Reduce heat and simmer, breaking up tomatoes with a spoon, 20 minutes. Stir in quinoa.

2. Heat remaining 1 tablespoon plus 1½ teaspoons oil in a large nonstick skillet over medium. Fry eggs to desired doneness, 3 to 5 minutes.

3. Serve soup topped with egg and thyme, and serve with hot sauce.

PER SERVING: *330 calories, 15 g protein, 31 g carbohydrates (5 g fiber), 16 g fat*

⫘→ PROTEIN BOOST

Add 1 (15-ounce) can white beans, drained, to the soup along with the tomatos. Top each serving with 2 tablespoons toasted pine nuts.

Sweet Potato and Black Bean Soup

SERVES 4

WHAT YOU'LL NEED:

2 TBSP OLIVE OIL

1 SWEET POTATO, PEELED AND DICED

1 ONION, FINELY CHOPPED

2 LARGE GARLIC CLOVES, FINELY CHOPPED

1 TBSP CHILI POWDER

4 CUPS LOW-SODIUM CHICKEN OR VEGETABLE BROTH

2 (15.5 OZ) CANS BLACK BEANS, RINSED AND DRAINED

1 AVOCADO, PITTED, PEELED, AND DICED

SLICED RADISHES

FRESH CILANTRO LEAVES

¼ CUP SHREDDED CHEDDAR CHEESE

1. In a large saucepan over medium, heat the oil. Add the potato, onion, garlic, chili powder, and ½ teaspoon salt, and cook, stirring frequently, until aromatic, about 4 minutes.

2. Add broth and bring to a boil. Reduce heat and simmer until potato is tender, about 15 minutes. Stir in beans and simmer until heated through, about 5 minutes.

3. Serve in bowls and top with avocado, radishes, cilantro, and cheese.

PER SERVING: *411 calories, 16 g protein, 54 g carbohydrates (19 g fiber), 18 g fat*

||⊢→ **PROTEIN BOOST**

Top each serving with 2 tablespoons each Greek yogurt and hemp hearts.

IT'S NOT A YAM, MA'AM

Sweet potatoes aren't really a potato at all. They're a type of morning glory—a tropical vine thats tuberous roots can be white, yellow, orange, red, purple, or brown. And they're not yams, either—even though they're often labeled that way in the grocery store. An actual yam is a starchy tropical vegetable that takes 8 to 11 months of warm weather to mature. They're very rarely found in North America.

The Plant Protein A-List

Legume: It's a weird word, but an important one if you're looking to eat more plants without sacrificing protein. Bone up for more muscle.

In general, beans and lentils are high in fiber (11 grams of protein in 1 cup kidney beans, and lentils have about 16 grams of belly-filling fiber in every cup), which is critical for maintaining a healthy weight, a hardworking heart, a good daily constitution, and slowing digestion. They're also high in antioxidants, B vitamins, iron, magnesium, potassium, copper, and zinc. Choose dried (soak and cook before use) or ready-to-eat canned.

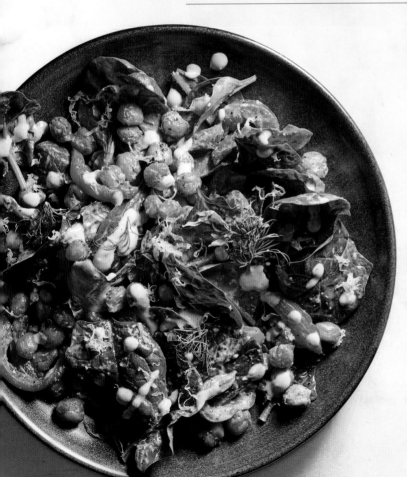

1 CHICKPEAS

▶WHAT IT IS
Chickpeas (a.k.a. garbanzo beans) are a legume, high in protein and fiber, and contain every amino acid necessary for muscle growth.

▶HOW IT TASTES
They have a mildly nutty flavor, buttery texture, and take on the flavor of whatever seasoning you're using. Roast for a crunchy snack, or toss into salads or soups.

PER ½ CUP COOKED: *355 calories, 20 g protein, 61 g carbohydrates (18 g fiber), 6 g fat*

COOK IT: *60 minutes*

2 KIDNEY BEANS

▶WHAT IT IS
These beans are an excellent source of thiamin and riboflavin, which help your body use energy efficiently. Plus, they contain 14 grams of cholesterol-fighting fiber per cup.

▶HOW IT TASTES
Kidney beans have a slight sweetness and a meaty texture. Throw them into chili, a wrap, or a salad—or whip up some Cajun-style red beans and rice.

PER ½ CUP COOKED: *300 calories, 21 g protein, 55 g carbohydrates (23 g fiber), 1 g fat*

COOK IT: *45 to 60 minutes*

3 EDAMAME

▶ **WHAT IT IS**
Edamame are young green soybeans. They're a great source of complete protein, fiber, and iron. Some studies suggest they have the power to lower cholesterol.

▶ **HOW IT TASTES**
Most often steamed or boiled, edamame have a nutty, fresh flavor and tender-crisp texture. Pop a bag of edamame in the pod in the microwave, then toss with toasted sesame oil and salt.

PER ½ CUP COOKED: 45 calories, 9 g protein, 8 g carbohydrates (4 g fiber), 4 g fat

COOK IT: 5 minutes

4 BLACK BEANS

▶ **WHAT IT IS**
Beans with darker seed coats have the most antioxidants—which earns this variety top marks. They're the only bean that boosts your brain power, from antioxidant compounds called anthocyanins.

▶ **HOW IT TASTES**
Black beans have a mild flavor and smooth, creamy texture from their white centers. Their subtle flavor makes them highly versatile for using in all kinds of dishes.

PER ½ CUP COOKED: 120 calories, 8 g protein, 20 g carbohydrates (9 g fiber), 0 g fat

COOK IT: 60 to 90 minutes

5 PEAS

▶ **WHAT IT IS**
They're legumes, which are technically beans, but let's not get into that. English peas are small but mighty. One cup offers up more than half of your daily value of vitamin K.

▶ **HOW IT TASTES**
The secret to maintaining their bright green color and sweet flavor is to cook them as little as possible—your choice to steam, boil, saute, or stir-fry.

PER ½ CUP COOKED: 45 calories, 2 g protein, 3 g carbohydrates (1 g fiber), 3 g fat

COOK IT: 2 to 3 minutes

6 BROWN LENTILS

▶ **WHAT IT IS**
The most common variety of lentil, they range in color from khaki-brown to dark black and make a flavorful filling substitute for refried beans.

▶ **HOW IT TASTES**
The lighter brown varieties (Spanish Brown, German Brown, or Indian Brown) have a mild, earthy flavor; the darkest variety (Beluga) have a rich and deep flavor.

PER ½ CUP COOKED: 115 calories, 9 g protein, 20 g carbohydrates (8 g fiber), 0 g fat

COOK IT: 20 to 30 minutes

7 GREEN LENTILS

▶ **WHAT IT IS**
Classified according to their size—large may be Laird, medium Richlea, and small Eston—green lentils are slate-green in color with blue-black undertones.

▶ **HOW IT TASTES**
This peppery-tasting lentil keeps a firm texture when cooked, making them ideal for salads or side dishes mixed with grains (think quinoa-lentil pilaf—yum).

PER ½ CUP COOKED: 140 calories, 12 g protein, 23 g carbohydrates (9 g fiber), 0 g fat

COOK IT: about 45 minutes

8 RED LENTILS

▶ **WHAT IT IS**
Red lentils range in color from gold to orange to, well, red. They're most commonly found in Indian curry dishes, like dal.

▶ **HOW IT TASTES**
Sweet and nutty, red lentils tend to lose their shape and get mushy when cooked, so this variety works well in curries and soups in need of thickening.

PER ½ CUP COOKED: 150 calories, 12 g protein, 26 g carbohydrates (2 g fiber), 0 g fat

COOK IT: about 30 minutes

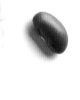

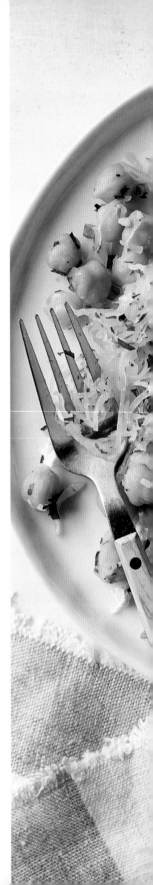

Sides

Old way of eating vegetables: Pop a meager salad on the side and drown it in dressing. New way of eating vegetables: Make that salad really, really delicious— so delicious that it becomes crave-able and impossible to ignore. Here are a handful of plant-based sides that are anything but unforgettable.

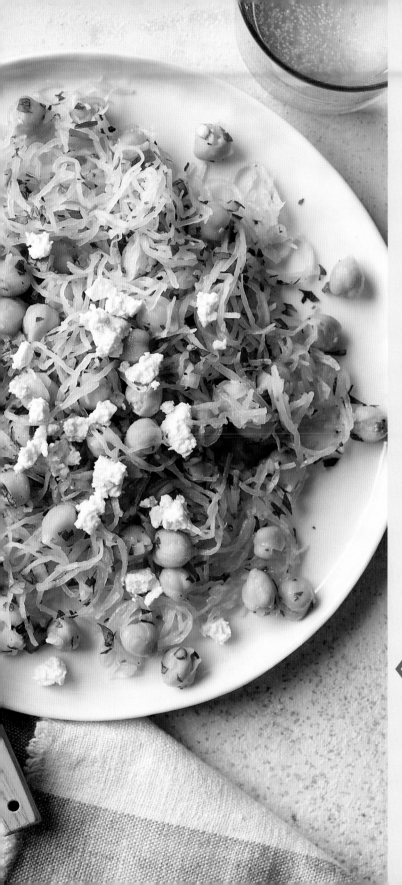

THE RECIPES

Charred Green Beans with Roasted and Hot Peppers

SERVES 2

WHAT YOU'LL NEED:

2 TBSP OLIVE OIL

¾ LB GREEN BEANS

1 ROASTED RED PEPPER, SLICED

6 PEPPADEWS, SLICED

¼ CUP PINE NUTS, TOASTED

1. In a cast-iron skillet (or other heavy skillet) over medium-high, heat the oil. Add green beans and cook until charred, 5 to 7 minutes.

2. Transfer to a plate and top with the roasted pepper, Peppadews, pine nuts, salt, and pepper. Serve hot or cold.

PER SERVING: *304 calories, 5 g protein, 17 g carbohydrates (6 g fiber), 26 g fat*

A PEPPA WHAT?

African Peppadew peppers are as much a brand as they are a variety. A South African man named Johan Steenkamp discovered these sweet piquanté peppers growing at his vacation home in the Eastern Cape. Peppadews are bright red cherry-tomato-size fruits with a crisp texture and a touch of sweetness that balances the burn. Most often pickled in brine, the peppers range in heat level, but the hottest aren't any hotter than a pickled jalapeño.

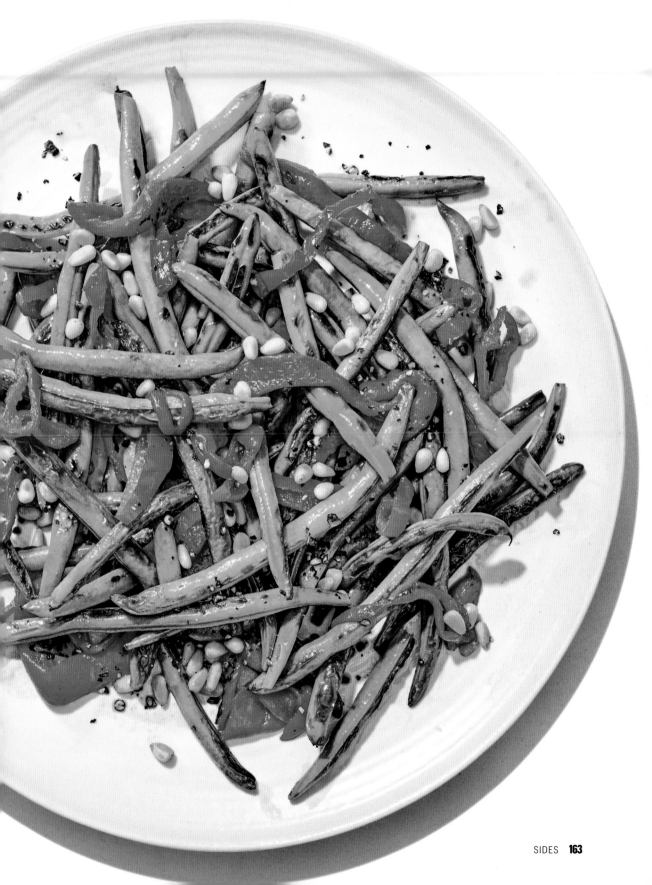

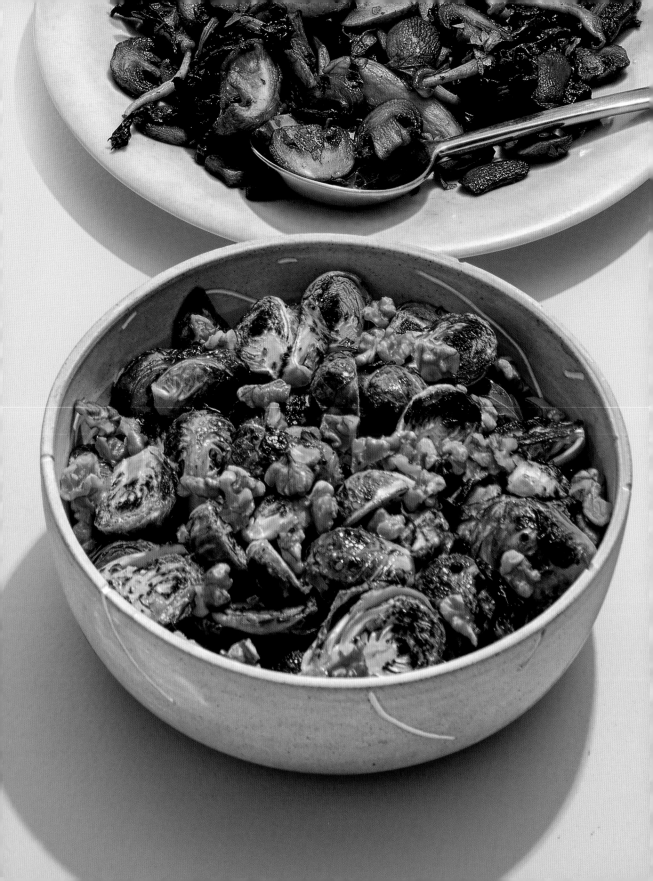

Charred Honey-Orange Walnut Brussels Sprouts

SERVES 4

WHAT YOU'LL NEED:

- 1 LB BRUSSELS SPROUTS, TRIMMED AND HALVED
- ¼ CUP OLIVE OIL
- 2 TBSP HONEY
- ZEST FROM 1 ORANGE PLUS JUICE FROM ½ ORANGE
- 1 CUP CHOPPED WALNUTS

1. In a large bowl, toss the Brussels sprouts, olive oil, honey, orange zest, and a pinch each of salt and pepper.

2. Heat a cast-iron skillet (or other heavy skillet) over medium-high, then add the Brussels sprouts. Cook until crisp-tender and charred, 6 to 8 minutes. Add the orange juice and walnuts and cook until glazed, about 1 minute. Season with salt and pepper.

PER SERVING: *375 calories, 8 g protein, 23 g carbohydrates (6 g fiber), 31 g fat*

THE SCIENCE OF SPROUTS

The small but mighty sprout is packed with fiber, folate, potassium, and vitamin C. Scientists have linked eating brassica vegetables that are rich in glucosinolates—such as cabbage, cauliflower, and sprouts—to pumped-up muscle gain. These compounds help stimulate the development of stem cells in your muscles, helping them to repair and grow.

Crispy Potatoes with Vegan Nacho Sauce

SERVES 4

WHAT YOU'LL NEED

- 2 LB MIXED BABY POTATOES, HALVED
- 3 TBSP CANOLA OIL
- 1 CUP UNSALTED RAW CASHEWS, SOAKED OVERNIGHT AND DRAINED
- JUICE FROM 1½ LEMONS
- ½ TSP CHILI POWDER
- ½ TSP GROUND CUMIN
- ½ TSP SWEET PAPRIKA
- ½ TSP GARLIC POWDER
- ¼ CUP NUTRITIONAL YEAST
- ½ JALAPEÑO, SEEDED AND CHOPPED

1. Preheat your oven to 450°F. Toss potatoes with canola oil, ½ teaspoon salt and ¼ teaspoon pepper. On a rimmed baking sheet, spread potatoes in a single layer. Roast until golden and crispy, stirring once, about 30 minutes.

2. Meanwhile, in a blender, puree cashews, lemon juice, chili powder, cumin, paprika, garlic powder, 1 teaspoon coarse sea salt, nutritional yeast, and jalapeño with 1 cup water until smooth. Transfer to a saucepan and heat over medium-low, stirring occasionally, until warm, 5 minutes. Transfer to a bowl and serve with the roasted potatoes.

PER SERVING: *380 calories, 10 g protein, 47 g carbohydrates (6 g fiber), 18 g fat*

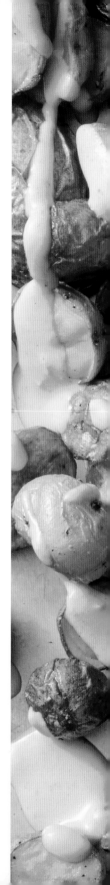

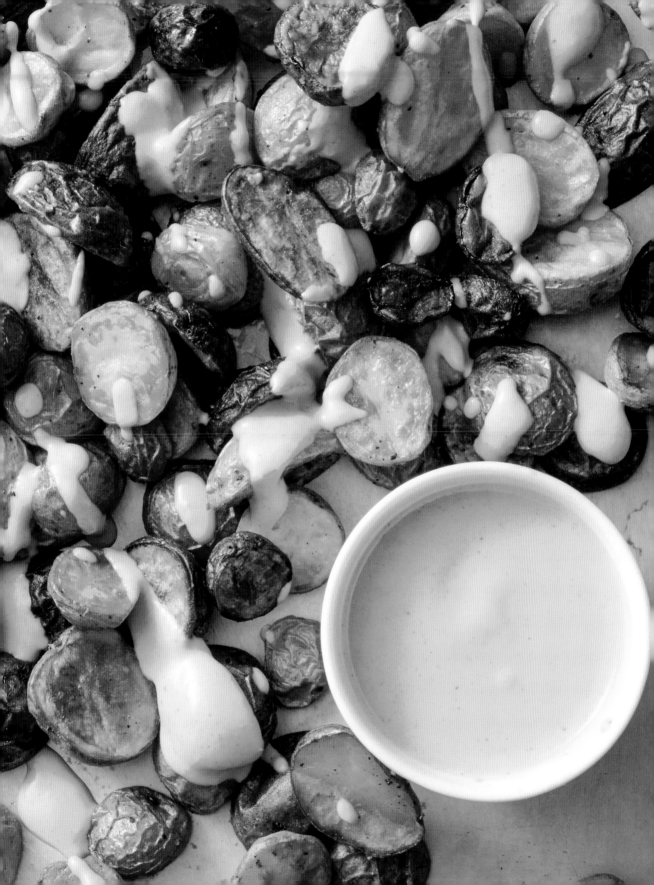

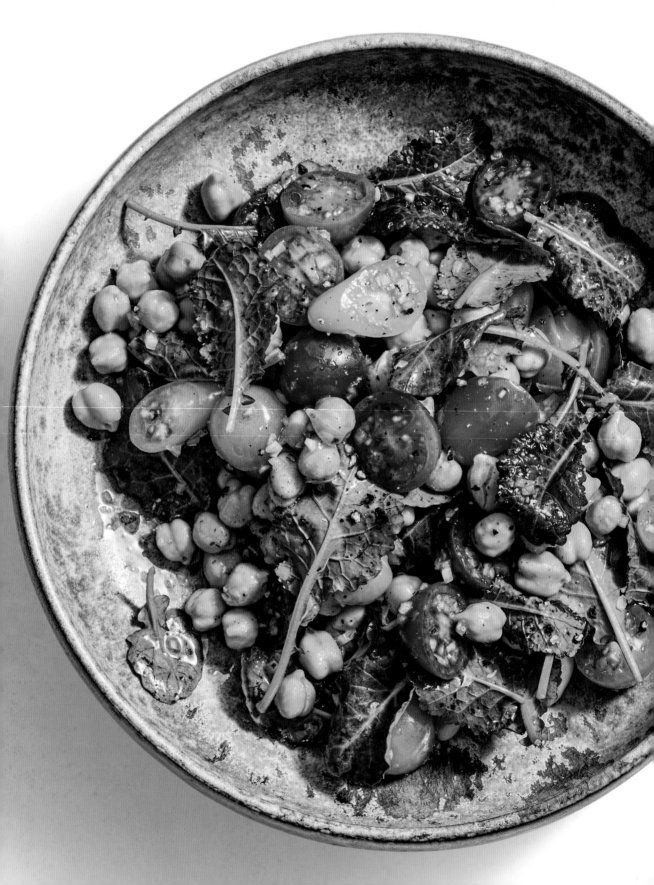

Kale, Cherry Tomato, and Chickpea Salad

SERVES 4

WHAT YOU'LL NEED:

- 1 (29 OZ) CAN CHICKPEAS, RINSED AND DRAINED
- 1 MEDIUM SHALLOT, MINCED
- 1½ CUPS CHERRY TOMATOES, HALVED
- 1½ CUPS PACKED BABY KALE
- 1 TBSP OLIVE OIL
- 1 TBSP WHITE WINE VINEGAR

In a large bowl, combine chickpeas, shallot, cherry tomatoes, baby kale, olive oil, vinegar, and salt and pepper to taste. Let the salad stand 30 minutes before serving.

PER SERVING: *257 calories, 11 g protein, 43 g carbohydrates (11 g fiber), 5 g fat*

WHICH OLIVE OIL?

Olive oil is probably one of most nutritious foods on the planet. Research shows that the healthy fat may help your heart and improve your body's ability to absorb other nutrients. Choose extra-virgin olive oil that has a harvest date within a year. Light can degrade the quality of an olive oil, so avoid buying any brand in a clear bottle, and store it in a cool, dark place like a kitchen cabinet.

Vegetable Trio on Sweet Mash

SERVES 8

WHAT YOU'LL NEED:

4 LARGE SWEET POTATOES, PEELED AND CUT INTO 1-INCH CHUNKS

3 OZ PLAIN YOGURT

2 TBSP BUTTER

1 TBSP OLIVE OIL

1 BUNCH KALE, CHOPPED

12 OZ MINI SWEET PEPPERS, SLICED

3 CLOVES GARLIC, CHOPPED

1 (15 OZ) CAN PINTO BEANS, DRAINED

1 TBSP LEMON JUICE

1 TBSP WORCESTERSHIRE SAUCE

¼ CUP SUNFLOWER SEEDS

1. In a large pot of salted water over medium-high, add the sweet potatoes and bring to a boil, then reduce heat to medium. Cook, partially covered, until the potatoes are tender, about 10 minutes. Drain. Add the yogurt and butter; mash until combined.

2. In large skillet or pot over medium, heat the olive oil. Add the kale, sweet peppers, garlic, and ½ teaspoon salt. Cook for 10 minutes, stirring frequently.

3. Add the pinto beans, lemon juice, Worcestershire sauce, and ½ teaspoon pepper. Cook 1 minute. Serve over mashed sweet potatoes and sprinkle with sunflower seeds.

PER SERVING: *223 calories, 8 g protein, 30 g carbohydrates (5 g fiber), 9 g fat*

CUT KALE QUICK

Using your hands, strip the leaves from the stem by starting at the top of the leaf and pulling down toward the bottom of the stem. Toss the stems, stack the leaves, and chop or slice.

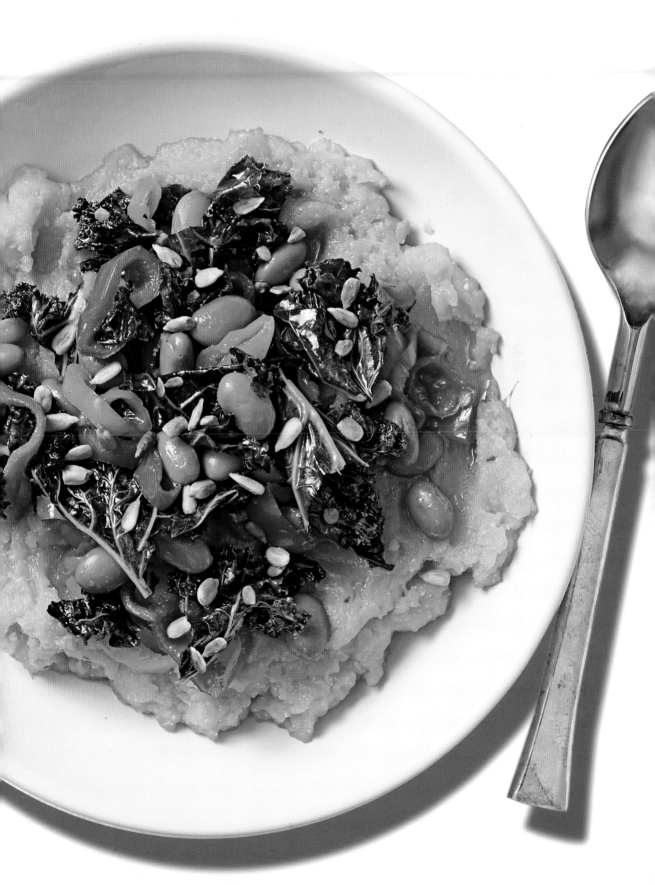

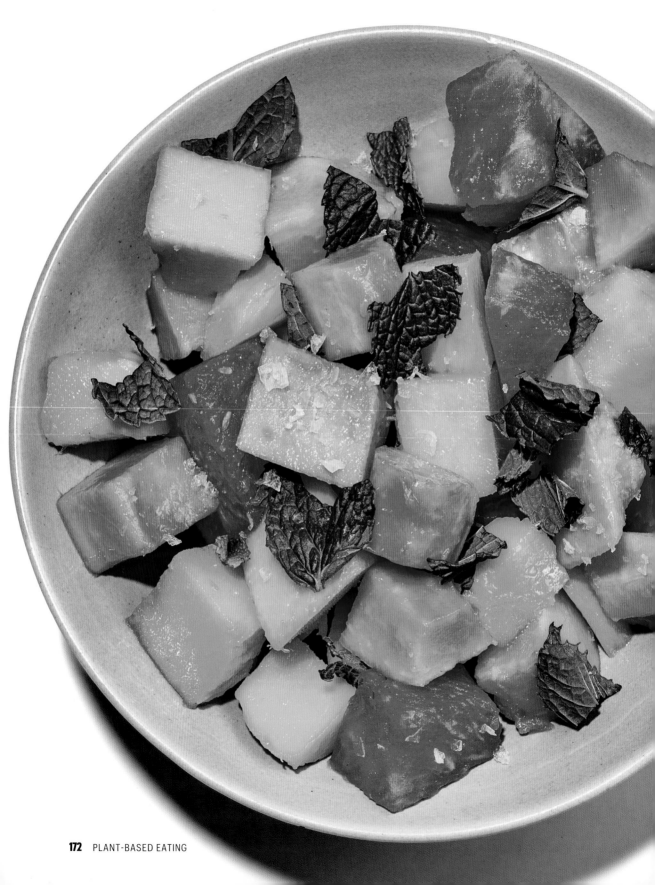

Tropical Fruit Salad

SERVES 4

WHAT YOU'LL NEED:

2 MANGOES, SEEDED, PEELED AND CUBED

2 GUAVAS, PEELED AND CUBED

2 PAPAYAS, SEEDS REMOVED, PEELED, AND CUBED

2 CUPS CUBED WATERMELON

¼ CUP FRESH MINT, CHOPPED

PINCH FLAKED SEA SALT

In a large bowl, combine mangoes, guavas, and papayas. Add watermelon, mint, and sea salt, and gently toss to combine.

PER SERVING: *213 calories, 3 g protein, 54 g carbohydrates (7 g fiber), 1 g fat*

QUICK-CUBE A MANGO

Stand the mango on one end and slice away the two thick sides of the fruit by running your knife down along both sides of the pit. Toss the pit. Place one mango half, skin side down, on the cutting board. Using a small sharp knife, cut a cross-hatch almost to the skin. Press the fruit from underneath to make the cubes pop up, then run a knife along the skin to cut the cubes from the skin and into a bowl. Repeat with the remaining half.

Apple, Arugula, Blue Cheese, and Walnut Salad

SERVES 2

WHAT YOU'LL NEED:

8 CUPS ARUGULA

2 APPLES, CORED AND DICED

¼ CUP CANNED CHICKPEAS, RINSED AND DRAINED

2 TSP OLIVE OIL

1 TSP BALSAMIC VINEGAR

2 TBSP CRUMBLED BLUE CHEESE

¼ CUP CHOPPED WALNUTS

In a large bowl, toss together arugula, apples, chickpeas, olive oil, and balsamic vinegar. Serve salads sprinkled with blue cheese and walnuts.

PER SERVING: *314 calories, 8 g protein, 36 g carbohydrates (8 g fiber), 18 g fat*

THE BIG APPLE

Not only are apples a good source of fiber, but they're also a rich source of disease-fighting antioxidants. If you've never found apples appealing, maybe you haven't tried the right apple right. Seek out Empire, Honeycrisp, Fuji, Pink Lady, or the orchard of other apple options out there ready for you to bite into.

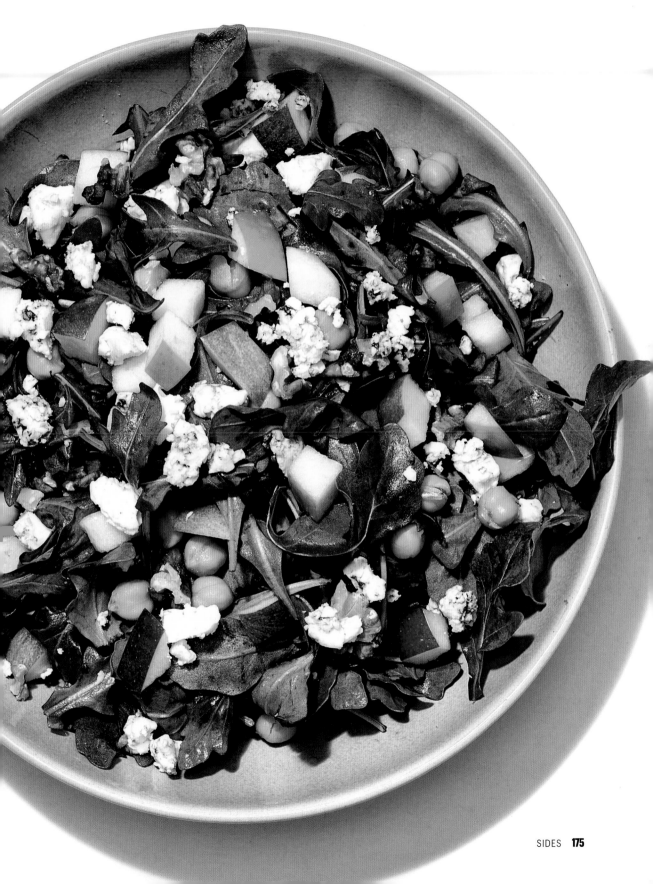

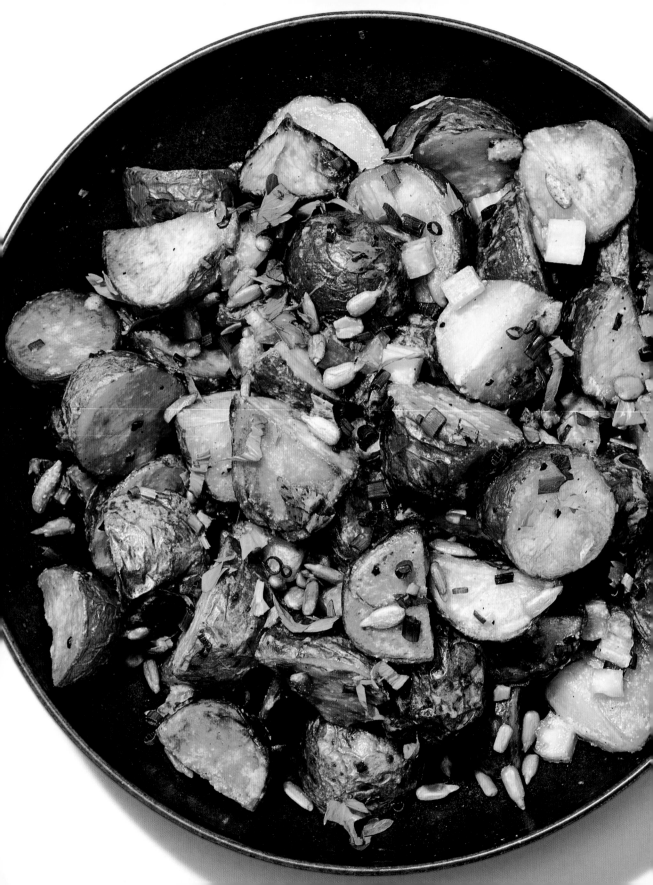

Dijon Roasted Red Potato Salad

SERVES 2

WHAT YOU'LL NEED:

- 1 LB BABY RED POTATOES, HALVED, OR QUARTERED IF LARGE
- 2 TBSP DIJON MUSTARD
- 2 TBSP CIDER VINEGAR
- 2 TBSP OLIVE OIL
- 2 STALKS CELERY, DICED
- ½ CUP ROASTED SUNFLOWER SEEDS
- 2 TBSP CHIVES

1. Preheat your oven to 375°F. Add the potatoes to a rimmed baking sheet and bake until browned and crispy, about 20 minutes.

2. Let cool slightly, then toss with the mustard, vinegar, olive oil, celery, sunflower seeds, and chives. Season with salt and pepper.

PER SERVING: *515 calories, 11 g protein, 53 g carbohydrates (8 g fiber), 30 g fat*

A NEW LEAF

Don't throw away your celery leaves. They're full of flavor, especially chopped up into quick vegetable-based salads like this one. Plus, because you already bought the stalked, celery leaves are free!

Three Bean Salad

SERVES 6

WHAT YOU'LL NEED:

1 (15 OZ) CAN CHICKPEAS, DRAINED AND RINSED

1 (15 OZ) CAN KIDNEY BEANS, DRAINED AND RINSED

1 (15 OZ) CAN BLACK BEANS, DRAINED AND RINSED

1 MEDIUM SHALLOT, MINCED

2 TBSP OLIVE OIL

1 TBSP RED-WINE VINEGAR

CHOPPED FRESH PARSLEY LEAVES

In a large bowl, combine the chickpeas, kidney beans, and black beans. Add the shallot, olive oil, and vinegar, and toss to combine. Season with salt and pepper, and sprinkle with parsley.

PER SERVING: *220 calories, 11 g protein, 33 g carbohydrates (10 g fiber), 6 g fat*

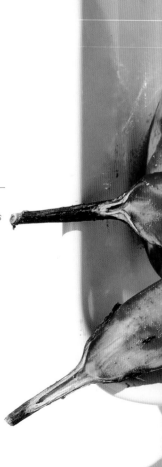

Gochujang Eggplant ❯

SERVES 4

WHAT YOU'LL NEED:

2 TBSP BUTTER

2 TBSP GOCHUJANG

1 TSP SOY SAUCE

4 JAPANESE EGGPLANTS, HALVED (OR 2 SMALL REGULAR EGGPLANTS, QUARTERED)

¼ CUP PEANUTS, CHOPPED

¼ CUP POMEGRANATE SEEDS

¼ CUP FRESH CILANTRO

In a small pan, melt the butter with gochujang and soy sauce. Preheat a grill to medium-high. Place eggplants on the grill and cook, uncovered, turning and basting with the butter, until charred, about 7 minutes. Cover and cook until tender, about 5 minutes. Top with peanuts, pomegranate seeds, and cilantro.

PER SERVING: *206 calories, 6 g protein, 25 g carbohydrates (9 g fiber), 11 g fat*

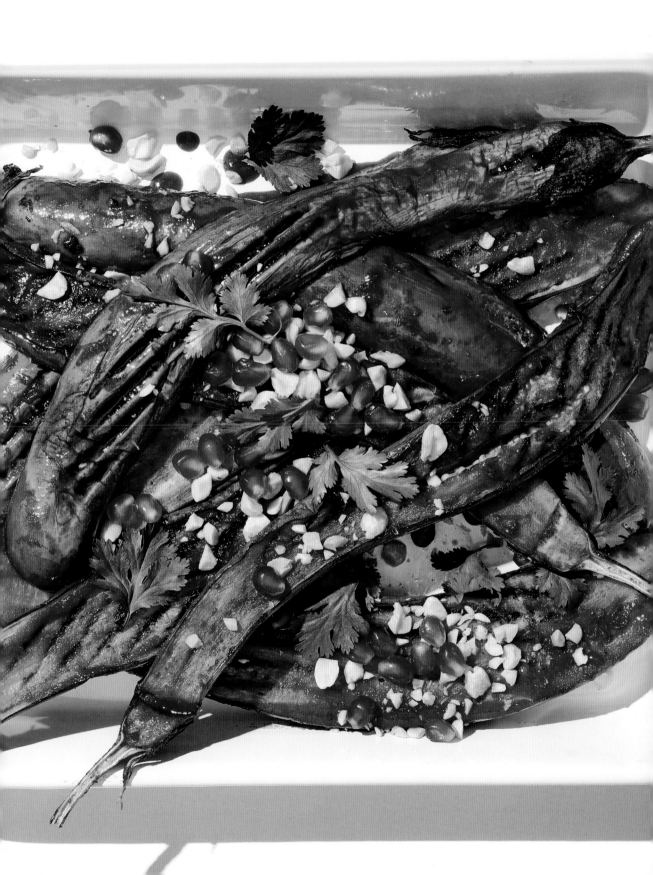

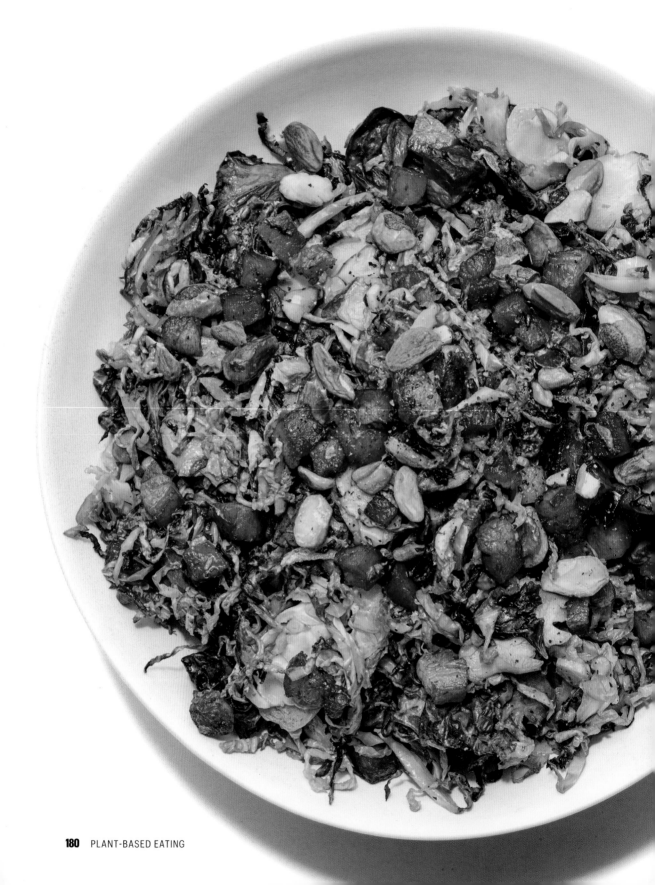

Shredded Brussels Sprouts with Pistachios and Prosciutto

SERVES 2

WHAT YOU'LL NEED:
1 TBSP OLIVE OIL
2 OZ PROSCIUTTO, DICED
1 LB BRUSSELS SPROUTS, FINELY SHREDDED
½ CUP UNSALTED PISTACHIOS

In a large pan over medium-heat, add olive oil, prosciutto, and Brussels sprouts. Cook until tender and slightly charred, about 8 minutes. Season with salt and pepper to taste. Transfer to a serving bowl and sprinkle with pistachios.

PER SERVING: *392 calories, 22 g protein, 30g carbohydrates (12 g fiber), 24 g fat*

GET SHREDDED

To prep Brussels sprouts for shredding, trim a very thin slice off the stem end of each sprout, then remove any loose outer leaves. Rinse well, then slice thinly with a sharp knife. If you have a food processor, you can use the slicing blade to make the process much quicker.

Berry and Wheat Berry Salad

SERVES 4

WHAT YOU'LL NEED:

- 1 CUP WHEAT BERRIES
- 1 CUP RASPBERRIES
- 1 CUP BLUEBERRIES
- ¼ CUP FRESH MINT LEAVES, FINELY CHOPPED
- 2 TBSP ROASTED SUNFLOWER KERNELS
- 1 TBSP BALSAMIC VINEGAR
- 1 TBSP OLIVE OIL

1. Cook wheat berries according to package instructions. Drain, transfer to a large bowl, and let cool to room temperature.

2. Mix wheat berries with raspberries, blueberries, mint, sunflower kernels, balsamic vinegar, olive oil, and salt and pepper to taste.

PER SERVING: *266 calories, 9 g protein, 44 g carbohydrates (10 g fiber), 8 g fat*

GRAIN GAINS

Research shows that three servings of whole grains a day can reduce risk of colorectal cancer by 17 percent. Whole grains also have high levels of antioxidants, some healthy fats, and vitamin E.

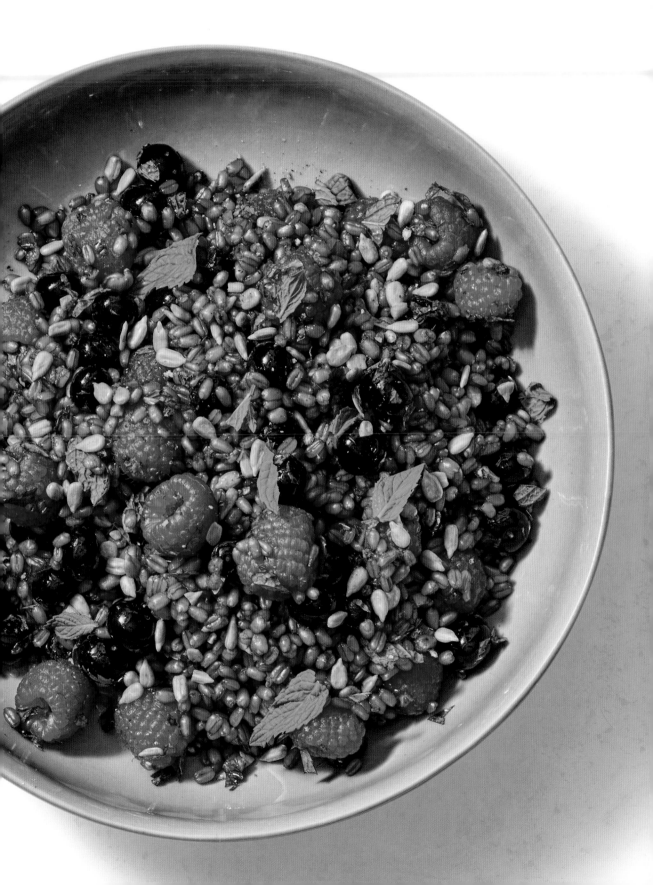

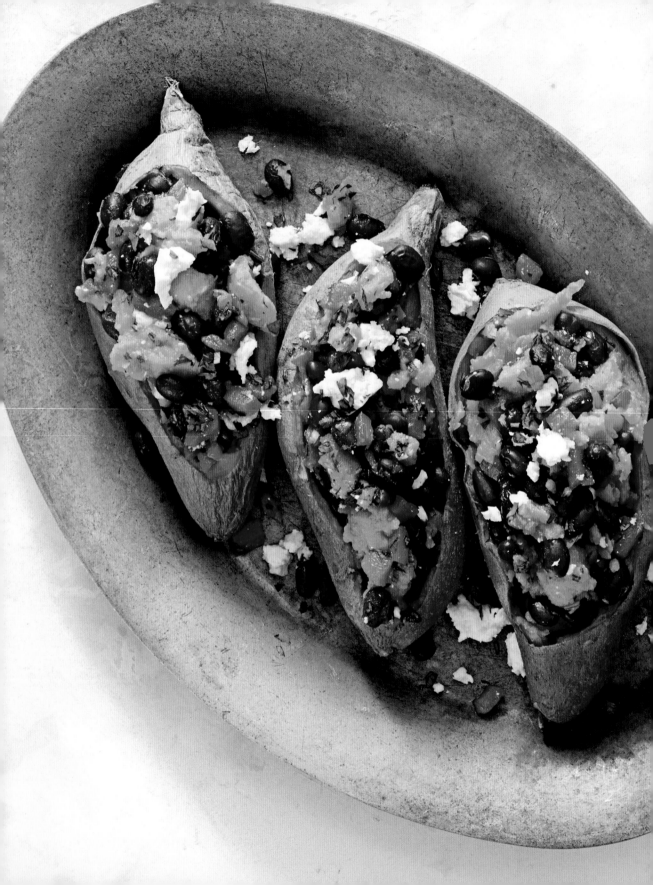

Loaded Sweet Potatoes

SERVES 4

WHAT YOU'LL NEED:

- 4 MEDIUM SWEET POTATOES
- 1 (15 OZ.) CAN BLACK BEANS, RINSED AND DRAINED
- ¼ CUP CRUMBLED FETA
- ¼ CUP ROASTED RED PEPPERS, FINELY CHOPPED
- 3 TBSP OLIVE OIL
- 3 TBSP FINELY CHOPPED FRESH PARSLEY

1. Preheat your oven to 400°F. With a small sharp knife, pierce the sweet potatoes all over, then arrange in a large microwave-safe baking dish. Microwave on high 10 to 12 minutes or until easily pierced with the knife.

2. In a bowl, combine the black beans, feta, red peppers, olive oil, parsley, and ¼ teaspoon salt.

3. Cut a thin slice from the tops of the sweet potatoes. With a fork, scrape sweet potato flesh to fluff, and place potatoes on a foil-lined baking sheet. Spoon black bean mixture onto each potato half, packing to fill. Bake until beans are heated through, about 10 minutes.

PER SERVING: *345 calories, 10 g protein, 50 g carbohydrates (13 g fiber), 13 g fat*

ROAST YOUR OWN PEPPERS

DIY roasted peppers taste way better than those from the jar. To make your own, wash the peppers well, halve lengthwise, and remove the stems and seeds. Arrange the peppers, cut side down, on a foil-lined baking sheet, and roast them in a 425°F oven until the skin blisters, 20 to 25 minutes. Carefully remove the peppers from the oven, cover with a sheet of aluminum foil and let stand for 15 minutes. When the peppers are cool to the touch, remove the skin, and store the peppers in an airtight container in the fridge for 5 to 6 days or freeze up to 2 months.

Spaghetti Squash and Chickpea Saute

SERVES 4

WHAT YOU'LL NEED:

- 1 3-LB SPAGHETTI SQUASH
- 1 SMALL RED ONION, FINELY CHOPPED
- 4 TBSP FRESH LEMON JUICE
- 1 TBSP OLIVE OIL
- 2 GARLIC CLOVES, CHOPPED
- 1 (15 OZ) CAN CHICKPEAS, DRAINED AND RINSED
- 2 TBSP OLIVE OIL
- 1 CUP LIGHTLY PACKED FRESH PARSLEY, FINELY CHOPPED
- 2 OZ CRUMBLED FETA

1. Using a large serrated knife, cut the spaghetti squash in half lengthwise; discard seeds. Place halves, cut sides down, on a parchment-paper-lined microwave-safe plate, and microwave on high just until tender, 9 to 11 minutes. Use a fork to shred squash strands. Transfer squash to a large bowl.

2. In a small bowl, combine red onion, lemon juice, and a pinch each of salt and pepper.

3. In a nonstick skillet, heat 1 tablespoon olive oil; add garlic and cook until beginning to turn golden brown. Add the chickpeas and cook for 2 minutes. Toss with the spaghetti squash, remaining 1 tablespoon olive oil, and ¼ teaspoon each salt and pepper. Fold in onion-lemon mixture and parsley. Top with feta.

PER SERVING: *245 calories, 7 g protein, 27 g carbohydrates (8 g fiber), 10 g fat*

CHECK OUT CHICKPEAS

Researchers in Canada have found that people who regularly consume chickpeas have healthier cholesterol levels than those who don't. Credit a high dose of soluble fiber, the kind that sucks up water, forming a gel in your intestines that blocks cholesterol. Soluble fiber may also fuel gut probiotics, the healthy bacteria that promote digestion, protect your colon, and give your immunity a boost.

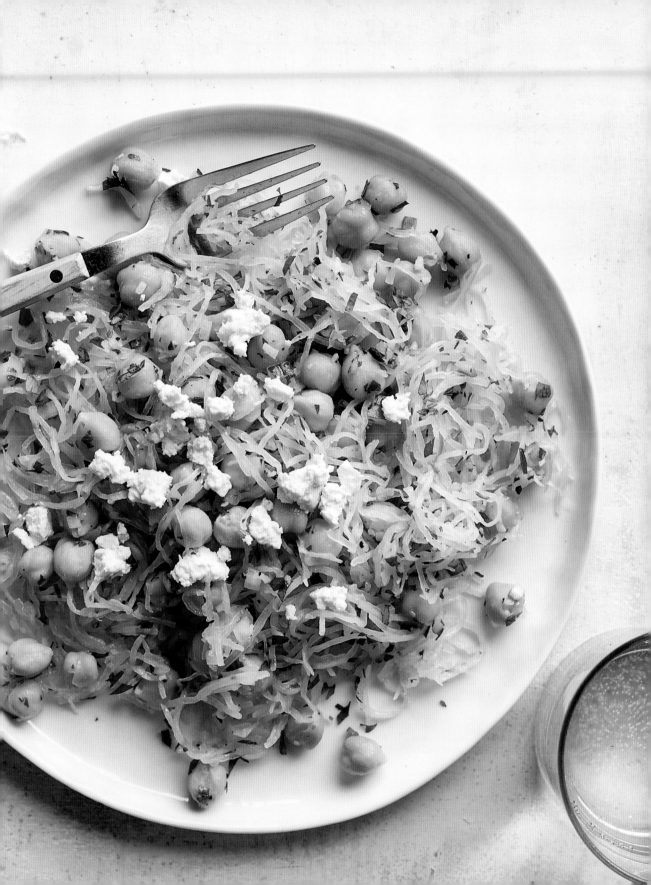

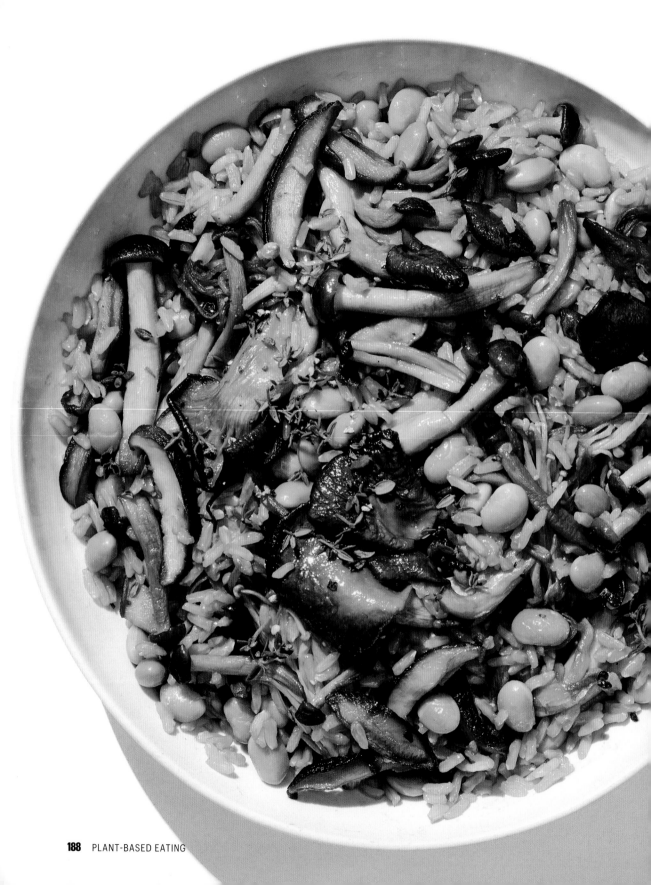

Mushrooms and Rice with Edamame

SERVES 6

WHAT YOU'LL NEED:

- 1¼ CUPS BROWN JASMINE RICE
- 1¾ CUPS VEGETABLE STOCK OR BROTH
- 2 TBSP CANOLA OIL
- 1 LB SLICED MUSHROOMS
- 1 CLOVE GARLIC, THINLY SLICED
- 2½ CUPS SHELLED EDAMAME, THAWED
- 1 TSP SOY SAUCE
- 1 TBSP FRESH THYME

1. In a medium saucepan, combine rice and stock and bring to a boil. Reduce heat to low and cook, covered, 40 minutes or until tender. Remove from heat and let stand 10 minutes. Fluff with a fork.

2. In a large skillet, heat oil over medium-high. Add mushrooms and cook until browned, stirring occasionally, about 10 minutes. Add garlic, edamame, soy sauce, thyme, and pepper to taste. Add rice to the skillet and carefully stir to combine.

PER SERVING: *285 calories, 12 g protein, 41 g carbohydrates (6 g fiber), 8 g fat*

FUN WITH FUNGI

Mushrooms are a key ingredient in a plant-based diet for their meaty texture and earthy flavor. Most varieties can be used interchangeably. Try regular white button mushrooms or cremini in this dish—or something more interesting, such as shiitake or oyster mushrooms.

Roasted Butternut Squash with Walnuts and Pomegranate Seeds

SERVES 4

WHAT YOU'LL NEED:

- 8 CUPS CUBED BUTTERNUT SQUASH
- 1 TBSP OLIVE OIL
- ¾ CUP CHOPPED WALNUTS
- ½ CUP POMEGRANATE SEEDS
- LEAVES FROM 2 SPRIGS FRESH THYME

1. Preheat your oven to 400°F. Toss squash on a rimmed baking sheet with olive oil. Season with salt and pepper. Roast until tender, about 20 minutes. Add the walnuts and roast until walnuts are toasted, 6 to 8 minutes more.

2. Transfer the squash and walnuts to a bowl and let cool slightly. Top with the pomegranate seeds and thyme.

PER SERVING: *292 calories, 6 g protein, 28 g carbohydrates (9 g fiber), 18 g fat*

IT'S THE POM

Fresh pomegranates are usually available from late September through December. Getting the seeds out of the fruit can be a bear, but you can often find the seeds—also called arils—in small containers in the refrigerated section of the grocery store. They're also available year-round in most frozen fruit sections. They take just minutes to thaw sitting out at room temperature.

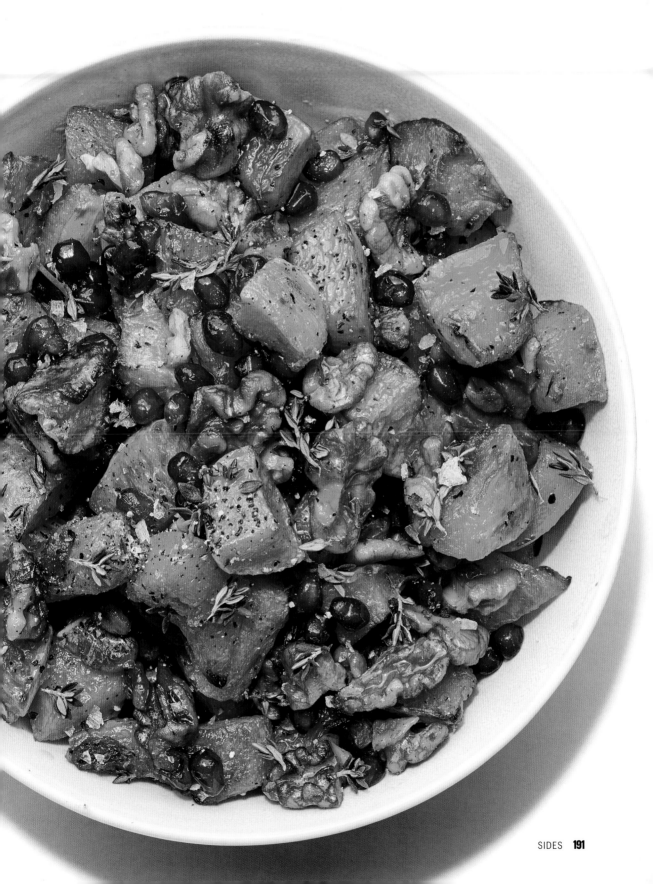

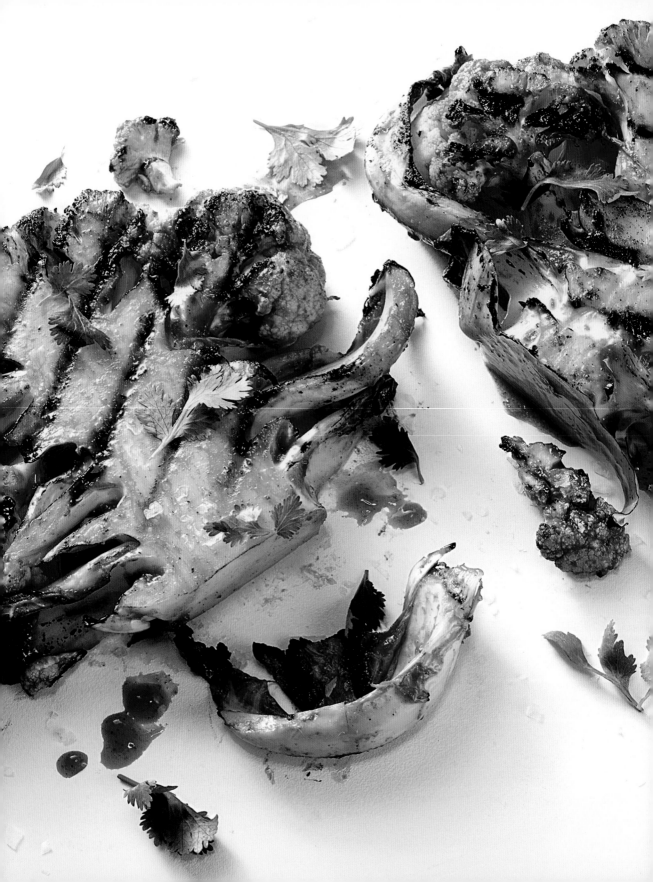

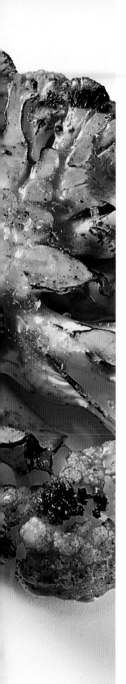

Cauliflower Steaks with "65" Sauce

SERVES 4

WHAT YOU'LL NEED:

2 TBSP KETCHUP

1 TBSP VINEGAR

1 TBSP SOY SAUCE

1 TSP HOT SAUCE

1 TSP CURRY POWDER

¼ TSP GARLIC POWDER

½ TSP CUMIN

½ TSP TURMERIC

1 LARGE HEAD CAULIFLOWER

1 TBSP OLIVE OIL

FRESH CILANTRO, FOR SERVING

1. In a bowl, mix the ketchup, vinegar, soy sauce, hot sauce, curry powder, garlic powder, cumin, and turmeric.

2. Starting from the center of the cauliflower, slice the head into four 1-inch slabs. Preheat an oiled grill or grill pan to medium-high. Brush the cauliflower slices on all sides with oil and season with salt.

3. Grill the cauliflower, covered, until tender, 5 to 8 minutes per side. Brush with the sauce and grill, uncovered, until blackened in spots, 2 to 3 minutes more per side. Top with cilantro.

PER SERVING: *98 calories, 5 g protein, 14 g carbohydrates (5 g fiber), 4 g fat*

DON'T 86 THE 65

The spicy and aromatic sauce for these grilled cauliflower steaks is inspired by the sauce for Chicken 65—a classic Indian appetizer of boneless deep-fried chicken coated in a fiery sauce that was invented in 1965 at the Buhari Hotel in the South Indian city of Chennai (formerly known as Madras). Theories abound as to how it got its name. One is that the sauce featured 65 different kinds of hot chilies, and of you were able to solider through a plate of it, you were *the* man.

The Great Grain Decoder

High in fiber and heart-healthy, whole grains are super, but there's nothing new about them. (Historians believe we've been eating them for about 10,000 years.) Here are six varieties you should get to know, and strategic tips for cooking them.

THREE WAYS TO COOK GRAINS BETTER

Don't rinse. Washing grains won't hurt texture or flavor, but it won't improve them either. Possible exception: quinoa. It's usually sold prerinsed, but check the package.

Be imprecise. Different grains call for different amounts of cooking liquid.

Easy fix: In a pot, cover dry grain with 2 inches of water. When it's done, dump the grain into a fine-mesh strainer to drain excess liquid.

Check doneness. Taste it from the pot. The grain should feel slightly chewy, not crispy or crunchy. Quinoa gives you a cue: when it's fully cooked, a curlicue pulls from each grain.

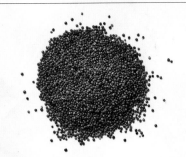

1 QUINOA

▶ **WHAT IT IS:**
This seed grows high in the Andes. Quinoa is gluten-free and has all nine of the essential amino acids, so it's a complete protein.

▶ **HOW IT TASTES:**
Properly cooked, quinoa has a texture that "pops." Its flavor is nutty and earthy. If you're making tabbouleh, try using quinoa instead of the traditional bulgur.

PER ½ CUP COOKED: *111 calories, 4 g protein, 20 g carbohydrates (3 g fiber), 2 g fat*

COOK IT: *12 to 15 minutes*

2 TEFF

▶ **WHAT IT IS:**
Teff has long been a culinary staple. This tiny poppy-seed-size grain is an excellent source of essential minerals, such as manganese, iron, and zinc.

▶ **HOW IT TASTES:**
The flavor depends on the color. Lighter teff will have a milder taste—almost like chickpeas. Darker teff tastes more roasty. It's good for adding bulk (and fiber) to meatballs.

PER ½ CUP COOKED: *127 calories, 5 g protein, 25 g carbohydrates (4 g fiber), 1 g fat*

COOK IT: *12 to 20 minutes*

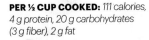

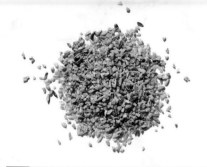

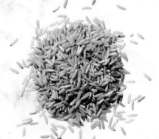

3 FREEKEH

▶ WHAT IT IS:
Farmers reap durum wheat before it's mature, sun-dry the seeds, and burn away the hulls. Freekeh can have more than double the protein and quadruple the fiber of brown rice.

▶ HOW IT TASTES:
Freekeh has a fire-roasted flavor and a texture that is dense and chewy, like brown rice. Cooked freekeh makes a tasty parfait base for Greek yogurt and fresh berries.

PER ½ CUP COOKED: *170 calories, 7 g protein, 33 g carbohydrates (8 g fiber), 2 g fat*

COOK IT: *20 minutes (cracked)*

4 FARRO

▶ WHAT IT IS:
This hearty stuff has been around since the Roman Empire. Farro is nutritionally similar to quinoa and a good source of fiber, protein, and calcium. Hail Caesar!

▶ HOW IT TASTES:
The texture is similar to that of brown rice, but the grain size is larger. Along with that comes a more pronounced nutty flavor. It's awesome when added to chili, stew, or soup.

PER ½ CUP COOKED: *200 calories, 7 g protein, 37 g carbohydrates (7 g fiber), 2 g fat*

COOK IT: *30 to 45 minutes*

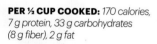

5 SPELT

▶ WHAT IT IS:
Spelt and farro are nearly the same in appearance. But spelt's tougher bran layer makes it better for grain-based salads, while farro is better for risotto and stews.

▶ HOW IT TASTES:
Spelt has a dense, chewy texture and the barest hint of sweetness. Freestyle a salad. Combine it with dried fruit, toasted nuts, and fresh herbs, plus oil, salt, and pepper.

PER ½ CUP COOKED: *123 calories, 5 g protein, 26 g carbohydrates (4 g fiber), 1 g fat*

COOK IT: *about 45 minutes*

6 BROWN RICE

▶ WHAT IT IS:
It's the supergrain from the 1970s, but still deserves to be on your table today. Processors remove the inedible outer hull but keep the nutritious bran and germ intact.

▶ HOW IT TASTES:
Compared with white rice, brown rice is denser, chewier, and nuttier. Mixed with some olive oil, salt and pepper, it's the perfect simple side dish with meat and fish.

PER ½ CUP COOKED: *124 calories, 3 g protein, 26 g carbohydrates (2 g fiber), 1 g fat*

COOK IT: *40 to 50 minutes*

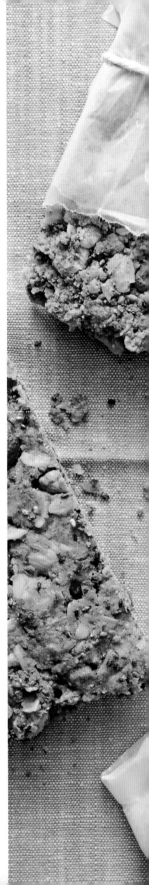

Snacks

Even when you're eating plant-based, snack attacks happen. So instead of going elbow deep in a party-sized bag of corn chips, turn to these easy hunger killers. They're easy to make as they are to eat.

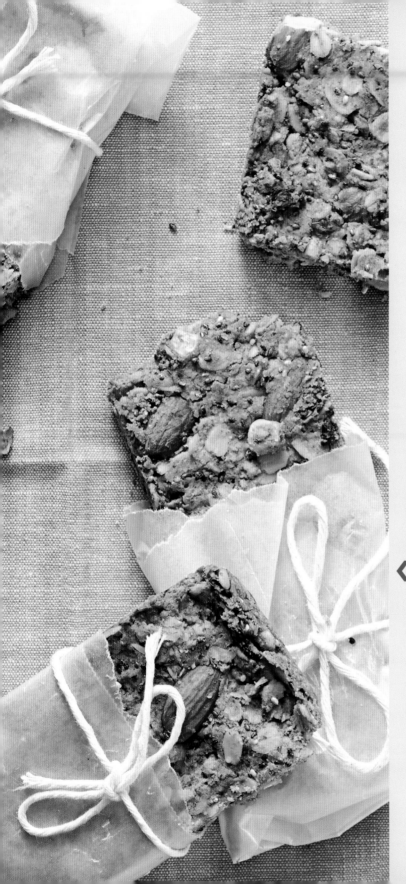

THE RECIPES

Sweet and Salty Maple Granola Bark

SERVES 12

WHAT YOU'LL NEED:

- ⅔ CUP PURE MAPLE SYRUP
- 2 TSP VANILLA EXTRACT
- ½ CUP OLIVE OIL
- 1 LARGE EGG WHITE
- 3 CUPS OLD-FASHIONED OATS
- 1 CUP SALTED ROASTED ALMONDS, COARSELY CHOPPED
- ½ CUP SUNFLOWER KERNELS
- ½ CUP ALMOND FLOUR
- 1½ TSP GROUND CINNAMON
- MILK AND FRUIT OF CHOICE, FOR SERVING

1. Preheat your oven to 350°F. Line a large rimmed baking sheet with parchment paper.

2. In a small bowl, combine the maple syrup, vanilla, olive oil, egg white, and ½ teaspoon salt. In a large bowl, combine the oats, almonds, sunflower kernels, almond flour, and cinnamon. Add maple syrup mixture to dry ingredients and mix thoroughly.

3. Use the back of a spoon to press the oat mixture evenly onto baking sheet. Bake until golden around the edges, 25 to 30 minutes, rotating pan once halfway through baking. Do not stir.

4. Let cool in pan on a wire rack 1 hour before breaking into chunks. Serve with milk and fruit. Store in an airtight container at room temperature up to 1 week.

PER SERVING: *335 calories, 7 g protein, 30 g carbohydrates (5 g fiber), 22 g fat*

SWEET SMARTS

Maple syrup is oozing with antioxidants—54 of them to be exact, 5 of which are unique to maple. Just be sure you select pure maple syrup. The other stuff—while much cheaper—commonly contains high-fructose corn syrup, artificial caramel coloring, thickening agents, and additives and preservatives such as sodium benzoate and sulfur dioxide. It's usually labeled "maple-flavor syrup" or "pancake syrup." Don't fall for it.

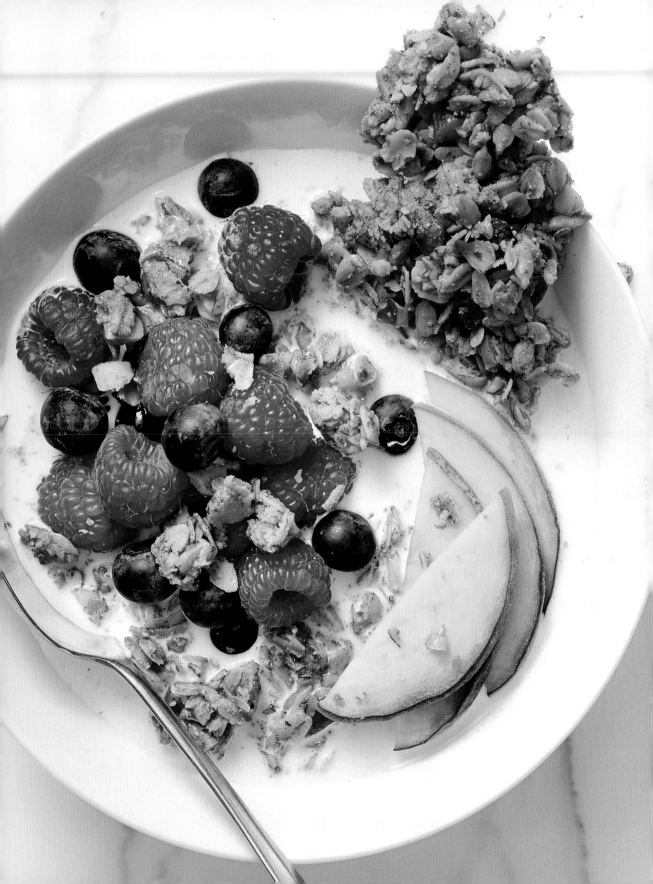

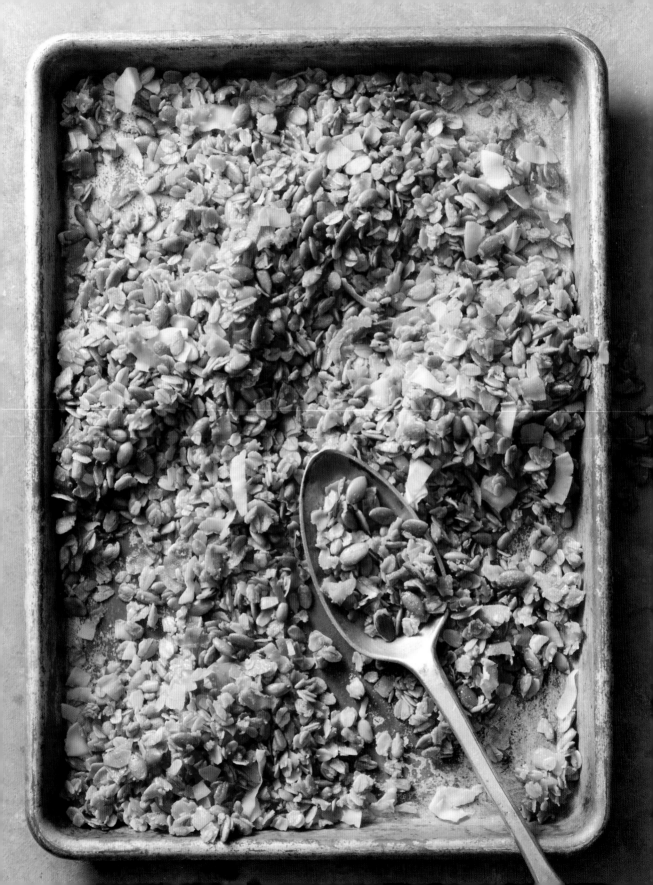

Best-Ever Granola

MAKES 7 CUPS

WHAT YOU'LL NEED:

½ CUP OLIVE OIL OR EXTRA-VIRGIN COCONUT OIL (MELTED)

¾ CUP PURE MAPLE SYRUP

2 TBSP TURBINADO SUGAR

3 CUPS OLD-FASHIONED ROLLED OATS

1 CUP UNSWEETENED COCONUT FLAKES

¾ CUP SUNFLOWER KERNELS

¾ CUP PUMPKIN SEEDS (PEPITAS)

1. Preheat your oven to 300°F. In a large bowl, combine the oil, maple syrup, sugar, and 1 teaspoon kosher salt. Add oats, coconut, and sunflower kernels, pumpkin seeds, and stir to coat.

2. Transfer to a parchment-lined baking sheet, spreading in an even layer. Bake, stirring every 15 minutes, until granola is light golden brown and dry, 45 to 55 minutes. Let cool completely.

PER SERVING: *305 calories, 6 g protein, 29 g carbohydrates (4 g fiber), 20 g fat*

KNOW YOUR OATS

There are three types of oats: steel-cut, rolled (a.k.a old-fashioned), and quick-cooking. Steel-cut oats—sometimes called Irish oats—are made from oat grains that are cut into two or three pieces with a steel blade. Rolled oats are made by steaming the grains and rolling them into flakes. Quick-cooking oats are made the same way as rolled oats—they're just steamed longer and rolled thinner to, well, cook more quickly. Old-fashioned rolled oats are the best choice for making granola because they hold their shape relatively well and the granola will have a crisp texture.

Paprika-Parmesan Granola Bars

SERVES 8

WHAT YOU'LL NEED:

1 CUP ROLLED OATS, TOASTED

½ CUP CRISP RICE CEREAL

½ CUP GRATED PARMESAN

½ CUP FREEZE-DRIED VEGETABLE BITS

⅓ CUP SMOKED ALMONDS, CHOPPED

3 TBSP CHIA SEEDS

½ TSP SMOKED PAPRIKA, GROUND CUMIN, CHILI POWDER, OR GARLIC POWDER

2 LARGE EGG WHITES, BEATEN

½ CUP PEANUT, ALMOND, OR CASHEW NUT BUTTER

1. Preheat your oven to 350°F. Line an 8×8-inch pan with foil, then grease the foil. In a medium bowl, combine the rolled oats, rice cereal, Parmesan, vegetable bits, smoked almonds, chia seeds, smoked paprika, ½ teaspoon each salt and pepper. Stir in egg whites and nut butter.

2. Press the oat mixture firmly into the pan. Bake for 30 minutes. Cool completely in the pan on a wire rack. Remove from pan and cut into 8 bars. Store in an airtight container at room temperature up to 1 week.

PER SERVING: *235 calories, 10 g protein, 18 g carbohydrates (5 g fiber), 16 g fat*

CHIA LATER

Studies have shown that chia seeds have cardioprotective properties and can help stabilize blood sugar. You can also sprinkle them onto salads, stir into yogurt or oats, or blend into your postworkout shakes.

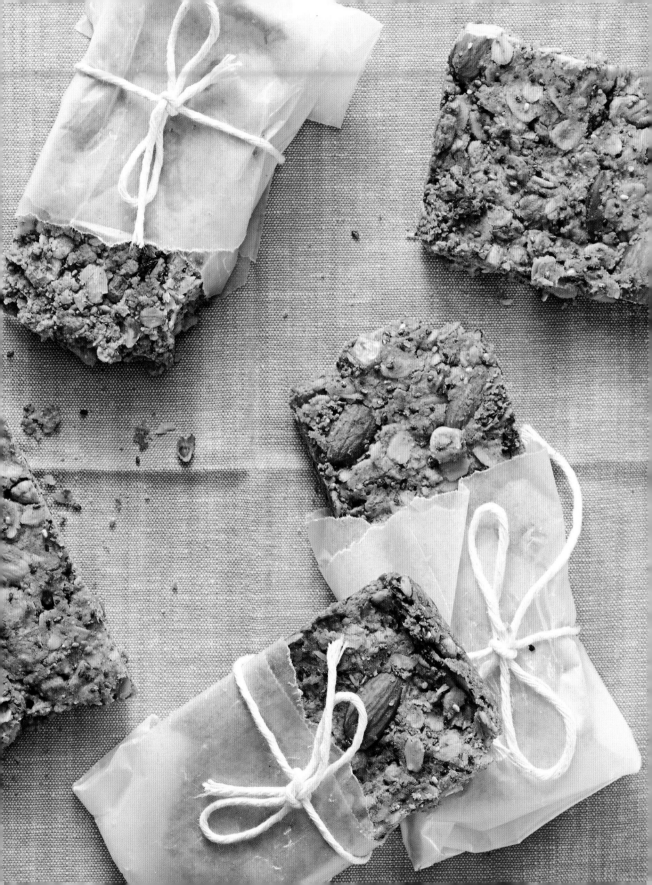

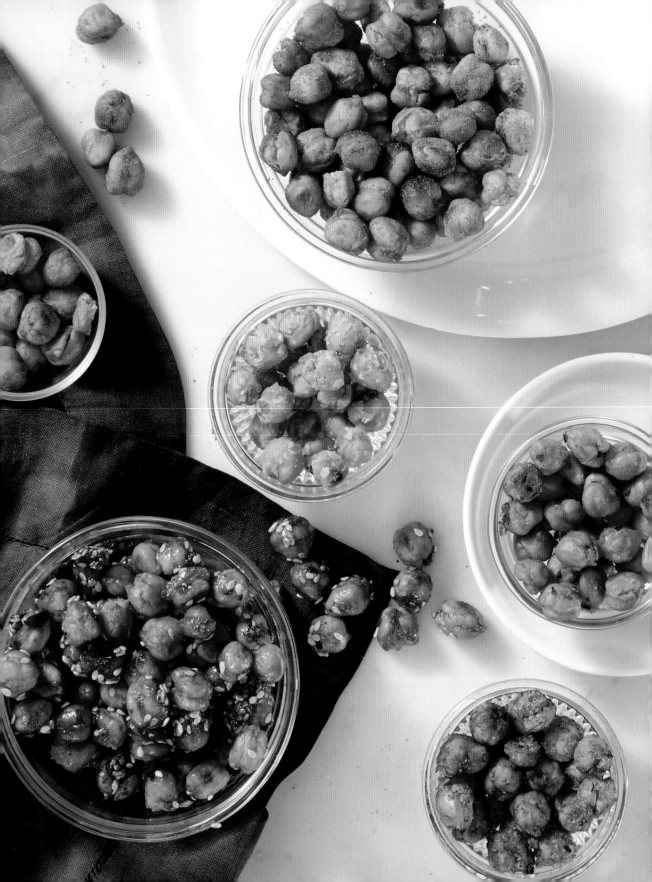

Chickpea "Nuts"

SERVES 8

WHAT YOU'LL NEED:

2 (15 OZ) CANS CHICKPEAS, RINSED AND DRAINED

2 TBSP OLIVE OIL

SEASONING OF CHOICE (RECIPES BELOW)

1. Preheat oven to 425°F. Pat chickpeas dry with paper towels, discarding any loose skins. On a large rimmed baking sheet, toss with olive oil, ¼ teaspoon each salt and pepper. Roast until crisp, shaking occasionally, 30 minutes.

2. Transfer chickpeas to a bowl; toss with desired seasoning, below. Chickpeas will continue to crisp as they cool. Makes about 2 cups. (If not eating right away, recrisp in a 350°F oven for 5 to 8 minutes.)

PER SERVING: *105 calories, 5 g protein, 15 g carbohydrates (4 g fiber), 3 g fat*

Freestyle on Flavor

BBQ
Toss roasted chickpeas with 1 teaspoon **dark brown sugar** and ½ teaspoon each **ground cumin, smoked paprika, garlic powder,** and **chili powder.**
PER SERVING: *126 calories, 5 g protein, 16 g carbohydrates (4 g fiber), 5 g fat*

Honey-Sesame
Toss roasted chickpeas with 2 tablespoons **honey;** 1 tablespoon each **sesame oil, sesame seeds,** and **sugar;** and ½ teaspoon each **garlic powder** and **five-spice powder.** Return to the oven for 5 minutes and bake until caramelized and crisp.
PER SERVING: *166 calories, 5 g protein, 22 g carbohydrates (4 g fiber), 7 g fat*

Maple-Cinnamon
Toss roasted chickpeas with 2 tablespoons **maple syrup,** 2 teaspoons **sugar,** 1 teaspoon **ground cinnamon,** and ¼ teaspoon **ground nutmeg.** Return to oven for 5 minutes and bake until caramelized and crisp.
PER SERVING: *140 calories, 5 g protein, 20 g carbohydrates (4 g fiber), 5 g fat*

Spicy Buffalo
Toss roasted chickpeas with ¼ cup **hot sauce.** Return to oven for 5 minutes and bake until dry and crisp.
PER SERVING: *122 calories, 5 g protein, 15 g carbohydrates (4 g fiber), 5 g fat*

Masala
Toss roasted chickpeas with ½ teaspoon each **garam masala, ground cumin, and ground ginger** and ¼ teaspoon **cayenne pepper.** Return to oven for 5 minutes and bake until dry and crisp.
PER SERVING: *123 calories, 5 g protein, 15 g carbohydrates (4 g fiber), 5 g fat*

Parmesan-Herb
Toss roasted chickpeas with ¼ cup **finely grated Parmesan** and 1 teaspoon each **garlic powder, finely chopped fresh rosemary,** and loosely packed **lemon zest.**
PER SERVING: *134 calories, 5 g protein, 16 g carbohydrates (4 g fiber), 6 g fat*

Chocolatey Clusters ❯

SERVES 4

WHAT YOU'LL NEED:

3 OZ BITTERSWEET CHOCOLATE, FINELY CHOPPED

2 TSP ESPRESSO POWDER

½ CUP WHOLE ROASTED ALMONDS

½ CUP CASHEWS

½ TO ¾ TSP FLAKED SEA SALT

1. In a saucepan over medium, melt chocolate with espresso powder, stirring until smooth. Stir in almonds and cashews until coated.

2. Transfer to a parchment-lined baking sheet, spreading in an even layer. Sprinkle with sea salt and chill until set. Break into pieces before serving.

PER SERVING: *317 calories, 8 g protein, 20 g carbohydrates (4 g fiber), 26 g fat*

Spicy Walnuts

SERVES 12

WHAT YOU'LL NEED:

¼ CUP SUGAR

2 TSP PAPRIKA

1 TSP GROUND CUMIN

½ TSP GROUND CINNAMON

1 LARGE EGG WHITE

1 TBSP HOT PEPPER SAUCE

3 CUPS WALNUTS

1. Preheat your oven to 325°F. Line a large rimmed baking sheet with parchment paper.

2. In large bowl, combine the sugar, paprika, cumin, cinnamon, 1½ teaspoons salt, and ½ teaspoon pepper. Stir in egg white and hot sauce until well combined. Add walnuts and toss to coat.

3. Arrange walnuts in a single layer on the prepared baking sheet. Bake, stirring once halfway through, until toasted and dry, about 25 minutes.

PER SERVING: *183 calories, 4 g protein, 8 g carbohydrates (2 g fiber), 16 g fat*

TRUST THE DARK SIDE

Research has shown dark chocolate can improve both heart health and blood pressure—likely due to its antioxidant content. But there's a caveat: The effects are with dark chocolate—70 percent and above.

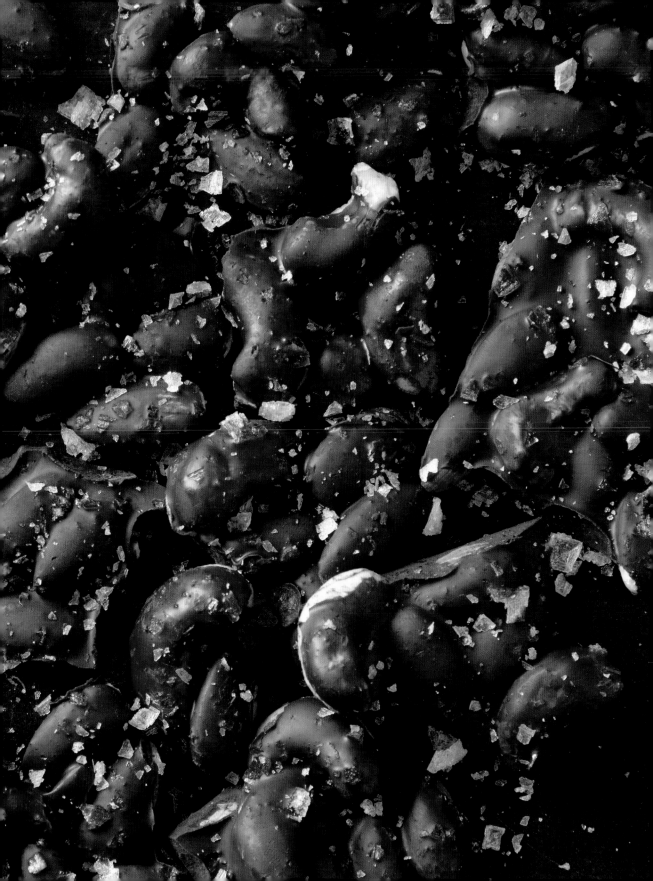

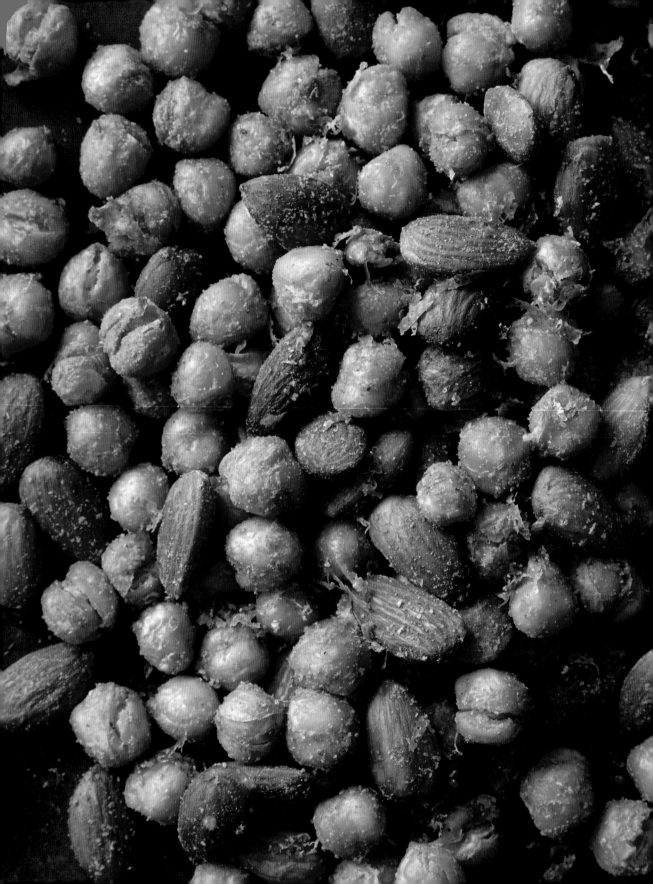

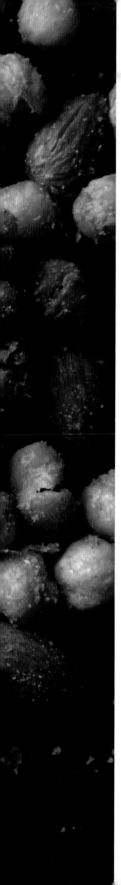

Curried Snack Mix

SERVES 4

WHAT YOU'LL NEED:

½ CUP CHICKPEAS, DRAINED AND RINSED

½ CUP WHOLE UNSALTED DRY-ROASTED ALMONDS

2 TSP COCONUT OIL

1½ TSP CURRY POWDER

½ TSP LIME ZEST

1. Preheat your oven to 375°F. In a medium bowl, toss the chickpeas with the almonds, coconut oil, and curry powder.

2. Transfer the mixture to a parchment-lined baking sheet, spreading in an even layer. Bake, stirring once, until golden brown, 15 to 18 minutes. Sprinkle with lime zest.

PER SERVING: *152 calories, 5 g protein, 8 g carbohydrates (3 g fiber), 12 g fat*

CURRY FLAVORS

There's no set recipe for curry powder—which is a blend of up to 20 spices, depending on the producer—but there are a few types that are widely available. The standard-issue yellow-gold blend is the most common and is usually mild, but it comes in hot varieties as well. The yellow hue is thanks to the spice turmeric. Madras curry powder is a blend that's typical of areas around the city of Chennai, India (formerly known as Madras). It has less heat than hot curry and less sweetness than mild curry. Any variety, works equally well here.

Wasabi Peanuts

SERVES 4

WHAT YOU'LL NEED:

- 1 EGG WHITE
- ¾ CUP RAW PEANUTS
- 1 TBSP + 1 TSP WASABI POWDER
- ⅛ TSP CAYENNE PEPPER

1. Preheat your oven to 300°F. In a medium bowl, whisk the egg white until foamy. Stir in peanuts. In a small bowl, whisk the wasabi powder, ¼ teaspoon salt, and cayenne pepper. Stir into nut mixture until coated.

2. Transfer to a parchment-lined baking sheet, spreading in an even layer. Bake, stirring once, until golden brown, 25 to 30 minutes.

PER SERVING: *170 calories, 8 g protein, 6 g carbohydrates (3 g fiber), 14 g fat*

MAKE YOUR OWN WASABI PASTE

Now that you have that jar or package of wasabi powder, you can make wasabi paste. Stir together 2 teaspoons of the powder with 1 teaspoon cold water until it's thoroughly blended. Cover the bowl with a tight seal and turn it upside down for 1 minute. (This helps contain the developing gases that improve the flavor of the paste and make it hotter.) It's that simple. The powder can be stirred into vinaigrettes or mayonnaise, or added to dips like hummus or guacamole.

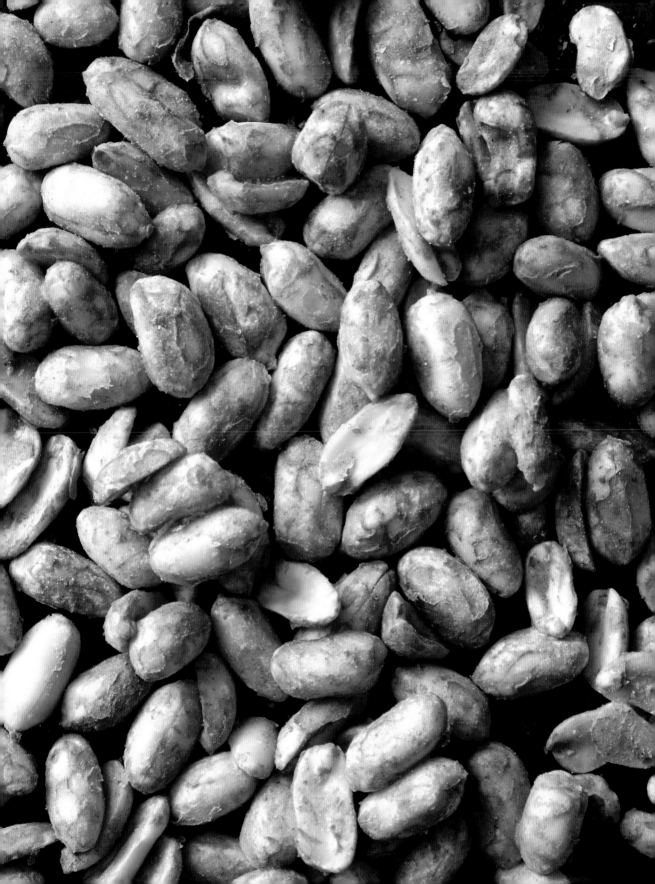

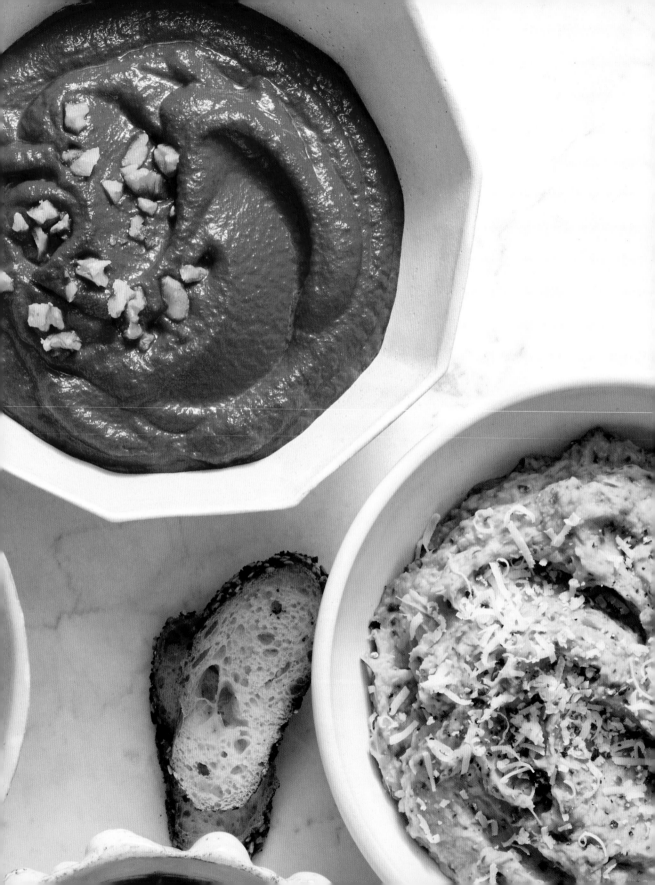

Zesty Beet Dip

SERVES 8

WHAT YOU'LL NEED:

8 OZ COOKED BEETS (ABOUT 5 SMALL BEETS)

⅓ CUP + 1 TBSP WALNUTS, TOASTED, DIVIDED

¼ CUP PREPARED HORSERADISH, SQUEEZED OF EXCESS MOISTURE

¼ CUP PLAIN GREEK YOGURT

1 TBSP FRESH LEMON JUICE

1 TBSP OLIVE OIL

1 TBSP WALNUTS

In a blender on low to medium speed, puree beets, ⅓ cup walnuts, horseradish, yogurt, lemon juice, oil, ½ teaspoon kosher salt, and ¼ teaspoon pepper until very smooth. Serve dip topped with walnuts.

PER SERVING: *115 calories, 3 g protein, 8 g carbohydrates (2 g fiber), 9 g fat*

Zucchanoush

SERVES 6

WHAT YOU'LL NEED:

1 LB SMALL ZUCCHINI (ABOUT 3), QUARTERED LENGTHWISE

3 TBSP OLIVE OIL, DIVIDED

1 CLOVE GARLIC

¼ CUP TAHINI

2 TBSP FRESH LEMON JUICE

3 TBSP FRESH MINT LEAVES, DIVIDED

FINELY SHREDDED PARMESAN CHEESE, FOR SERVING

1. Heat a grill to medium. Toss the zucchini with 1 tablespoon oil and ½ teaspoon kosher salt. Grill until tender and evenly charred, 8 to 10 minutes.

2. Transfer zucchini to a blender along with garlic, tahini, lemon juice, and 1 tablespoon mint; pulse to combine. On low speed, drizzle in remaining 2 tablespoons olive oil and puree until almost smooth.

3. Chop remaining 2 tablespoons mint. Serve dip topped with coarse pepper to taste and Parmesan.

PER SERVING: *125 calories, 3 g protein, 5 g carbohydrates (1 g fiber), 12 g fat*

Date and Nut Energy Balls

SERVES 16

WHAT YOU'LL NEED:

15 SOFT DATES, PITTED

½ CUP CASHEW BUTTER OR OTHER NUT BUTTER

½ CUP UNSWEETENED COCOA POWDER, PLUS MORE FOR COATING

2 TBSP FINELY SHREDDED UNSWEETENED COCONUT

1. In a food processor, puree dates, cashew butter, and cocoa powder until smooth.

2. Form into 1-inch balls and roll half in the coconut and the remaining half in more cocoa powder. Place on a plate or rimmed pan and refrigerate for 30 minutes. Store in refrigerator.

PER SERVING: *81 calories, 2 g protein, 10 g carbohydrates (2 g fiber), 5 g fat*

MEET YOUR DATE

There are hundreds of varieties of dates, but the most common (and available) are Medjool and Deglet Noor. Medjool dates are the larger of the two. They're moist and sweet, with skin that ranges from brown to black. Deglet Noor dates are smaller, drier, and firmer. They have a slightly nutty flavor. You'll want to be sure to use Medjool dates for these energy balls—they'll puree better and their moisture will help bind the ingredients together.

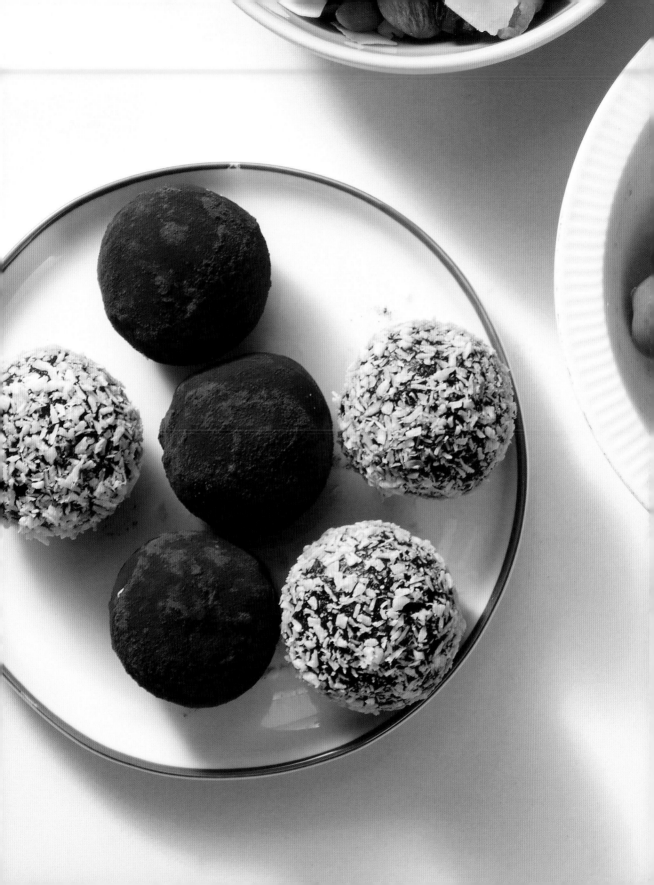

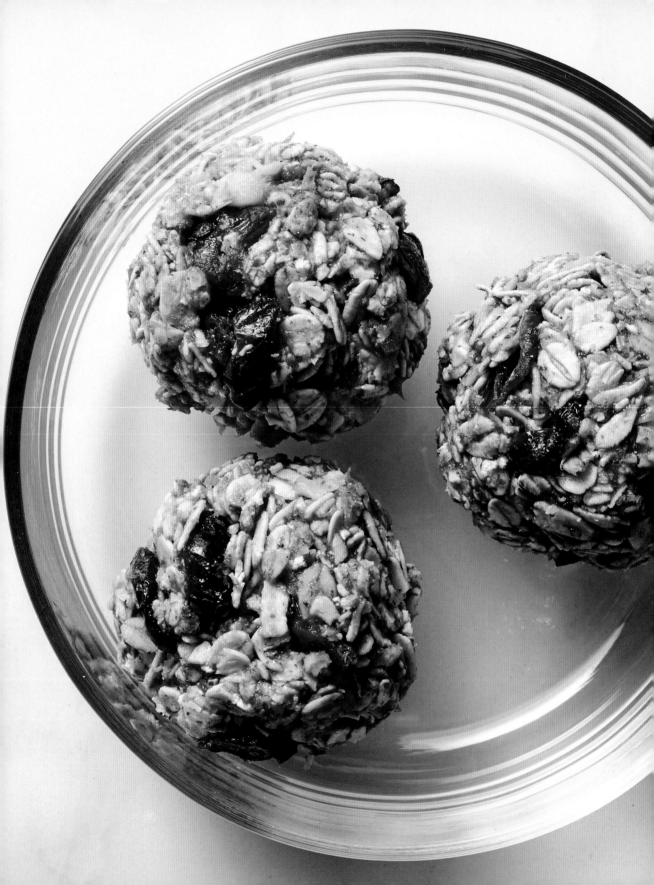

Peanut Butter and Cranberry Energy Balls

SERVES 12

WHAT YOU'LL NEED:

2 CUPS OATS

2 SCOOPS (70 GRAMS) PROTEIN POWDER

1 BANANA, MASHED

2 TSP GROUND FLAXSEED

¼ CUP DRIED CRANBERRIES

¼ CUP PEANUT BUTTER OR OTHER NUT BUTTER

In a bowl, mix the oats, protein powder, banana, flaxseed, dried cranberries, and peanut butter. Form into 12 balls.

PER SERVING: *123 calories, 8 g protein, 15 g carbohydrates (2 g fiber), 4 g fat*

PB FTW

Peanut butter is an incredible food and makes everything you pair it with taste better. Like other nut butters, it's high in fat and calories, but the good news is you get a lot for your 190-calorie investment. It's packed with protein, fiber, vitamins, minerals, and phytochemicals. Just read the label to watch for added sugar and vegetable oils. It should contain nothing but peanuts and maybe a bit of salt.

Index

HEARST
HOME

Copyright © 2020 by Hearst Magazine, Inc.

Cover design by Waterbury Publications, Inc.
Book design by Waterbury Publications, Inc.

Library of Congress Cataloging-in-Publication Data Available on Request

10 9 8 7 6 5 4 3 2 1

Published by Hearst Home, an imprint of Hearst Books/Hearst Magazine Media, Inc.

Hearst Magazine Media, Inc.
300 West 57th Street
New York, NY 10019

For information about custom editions, special sales, premium and corporate purchases: hearst.com/magazines/hearst-books

Printed in China

ISBN 978-1-950785-21-6

Photography Credits

Ted and Chelsea Cavanaugh, 162
Ted Cavanaugh, 40, 94, 95, 95, 104, 107, 108
Jamie Chung, 27, 110, 113
Ryan Dausch, 187
Dory Dawson, 164
Bryan Gardner, 54, 118
Michael Hedge, 23, 47, 58, 69, 93
Mike Garten, 24, 31, 43, 57, 65, 77, 80, 86, 99, 100, 114, 117, 124, 139, 143, 147, 148, 152, 155, 167, 168, 171, 175, 176, 183, 184, 199, 200, 203, 204, 212, 215
Getty / vaaseenaa, 6
Getty Images / Aleksandar Nakic, 12
Getty Images / bhofack2, 136
Getty Images / Dean Mitchell,
Getty Images / Eva-Katalin, 10
Getty Images / Fascinadora, 49
Getty Images / The Washington Post, 158
Sam Kaplan, 19, 70
Chelsea Kyle, 32, 35, 36, 44, 45, 45, 89, 131, 172, 180, 191
Marcus Nilsson, 83
Danielle Occhiogrosso, 96, 132, 140, 144, 28, 66, 151
Con Poulos, 53, 61, 127
Emily Kate Roemer, 135
Jeffrey Westbrook, 192
Rodale Books, 73
Romulo Yanes, 207, 208, 211
Shutterstock / Baibaz, 48
Shutterstock / Bonchan, 15
Shutterstock / Brent Hofacker, 103
Shutterstock / Hong Vo, 15
Shutterstock / ifong, 15
Shutterstock / LesiChkalll27, 79
Shutterstock / Natalia Lisovskaya, 8
Shutterstock / Peter Hermes Furian, 128
Shutterstock / Trexdigital, 15
Christopher Testani, 20, 74, 179, 188, 194, 195, 216
Waterbury Publications, Inc, 194, 39, 120, 121, 159
Jeffrey Westbrook, 192
Romulo Yanes, 207, 208, 211
Romulo Yanes, 207, 208, 211

Cover design, Waterbury Publications, Inc.
Cover photograph, Michael Hedge
Food styling, Lucy-Ruth Hathaway